Protein Supplements for Vegans

SOUTHERLAND | COPYRIGHT 2023

Introduction: Plant-Powered Protein for Vegans

In recent years, there has been an undeniable surge in the popularity of veganism as a lifestyle choice and dietary preference. As more individuals opt for plant-based diets, it has become increasingly essential to explore the nuances of vegan nutrition to ensure that individuals following this path receive adequate nourishment. Among the various macronutrients that make up a balanced diet, protein takes center stage as a topic of utmost importance.

The rise of veganism represents a profound shift in our understanding of food, ethics, and sustainability. It's a movement driven by compassion for animals, concern for the environment, and a commitment to personal health. Whether motivated by ethical, environmental, or health reasons, individuals are choosing veganism as a means to align their values with their dietary choices.

However, while a vegan diet offers a plethora of benefits, it also poses unique challenges, especially in meeting daily protein requirements. Protein, an essential nutrient, plays a pivotal role in maintaining overall health. It is the building block of life, responsible for the growth, repair, and functioning of every cell in our bodies. From supporting muscle development to maintaining strong hair and nails, protein is non-negotiable for optimal well-being.

For vegans, protein needs can be met through a carefully planned diet that includes a variety of plant-based protein sources. Yet, in the fast-paced world we live in, convenience often becomes a factor, leading many vegans to consider protein supplements as a way to bridge the nutritional gap.

Protein supplements have gained recognition as valuable tools for vegans to ensure they meet their daily protein requirements. While whole foods such as legumes, grains, nuts, and vegetables are fantastic sources of plant-based protein, there are situations where the convenience and versatility of protein supplements offer a practical solution.

This book will delve into the various aspects of protein supplementation for vegans, exploring the types of supplements available, how to choose the right one, and how to incorporate them into your diet effectively. We will also address common misconceptions and concerns surrounding protein supplements, providing you with the knowledge and confidence to make informed choices about your vegan nutrition.

Before we embark on this journey through the world of vegan protein supplements, let's set the stage by understanding the basics of vegan nutrition, protein requirements, and the crucial role protein plays in a vegan lifestyle. Together, we will explore the abundant plant-based protein sources that nature provides, laying a strong foundation for your successful adoption of plant-powered protein supplements.

As we progress through the chapters, you will gain insights into the diverse world of vegan protein supplements, discover delicious recipes and meal ideas, and hear inspirational stories of individuals who have embraced plant-based protein to achieve their health and fitness goals. So, whether you're a seasoned vegan looking to enhance your nutritional choices or a newcomer to plant-powered living, this book is your comprehensive guide to harnessing the power of protein to thrive on your vegan journey.

Understanding Veganism

Veganism is more than just a dietary choice; it's a lifestyle and philosophy that has garnered significant attention in recent years. Rooted in ethical, environmental, and health considerations, veganism involves a deep commitment to minimizing harm to animals and is driven by various core principles.

At its heart, veganism is a philosophy aimed at reducing animal suffering. Vegans avoid not only meat, dairy, and eggs but also non-food products like leather, fur, and cosmetics tested on animals. This stems from a belief in the intrinsic value of all sentient beings and a commitment to alleviate animal suffering.

Ethical considerations are paramount in veganism. Many vegans are motivated by the conviction that exploiting animals for food, clothing, or other purposes is inherently wrong. This ethical stance is based on the belief that animals should not endure harm, suffering, or death for human convenience or preference.

Environmental impact is another critical aspect of veganism. Aware of the significant resources required for animal agriculture, including land, water, and food crops, vegans are concerned about the greenhouse gas emissions and deforestation associated with the meat industry. They advocate for sustainable and eco-friendly food production.

Health and well-being are also driving factors for some vegans. Research indicates that a well-planned vegan diet can fulfill all necessary nutritional requirements, often leading to weight management, lower cholesterol, and a reduced risk of chronic diseases. A diet rich in whole, plant-based foods contributes to overall health.

Animal welfare and activism are integral to many vegans' lives. Engaging in animal rights activism, participating in campaigns, and raising awareness about animal treatment across various industries are common pursuits. Central to vegan advocacy is the goal of improving animal welfare and effecting positive change.

Nutritionally, a vegan diet focuses on plant-based foods like fruits, vegetables, grains, legumes, nuts, and seeds, providing essential nutrients like fiber, vitamins, and minerals. Vegans may need to be mindful of certain nutrients like vitamin B12, iron, calcium, and omega-3 fatty acids, obtainable through fortified foods or supplements.

Contrary to common misconceptions, veganism offers a rich diversity of culinary options. With global flavors and innovative plant-based alternatives developed by chefs and food companies, vegans can enjoy a wide range of foods, including plant-based burgers, dairy-free ice cream, vegan cheese, and meat substitutes.

The vegan movement is a growing global phenomenon, far from being a small, niche community. As awareness of the ethical, environmental, and health implications of dietary choices increases, veganism is becoming more accessible and mainstream.

The Importance of Protein in a Vegan Diet

Protein is an indispensable nutrient that plays a crucial role in the overall health and well-being of individuals, regardless of their dietary choices. In the context of a vegan diet, understanding the importance of protein becomes particularly significant, as it is often a topic of concern and curiosity. Let's explore why protein holds such a vital place in a vegan's daily nutrition.

1. Building Blocks of Life:

Proteins are often referred to as the "building blocks of life" for a reason. They are essential for the growth, repair, and maintenance of tissues throughout the body. Proteins are not just about building muscle; they are involved in creating enzymes, hormones, antibodies, and even the structural components of cells.

2. Amino Acids:

Proteins are made up of amino acids, which are the fundamental molecules that form protein structures. There are twenty different amino acids, and our bodies require all of them for various physiological processes. Nine of these amino acids are considered essential, meaning the body cannot produce them on its own and must obtain them from the diet.

3. Meeting Nutritional Needs:

In a vegan diet, it is entirely possible to meet all protein and amino acid requirements through plant-based sources. While animal products are rich sources of complete protein (containing all essential amino acids), vegans can achieve the same by consuming a variety of plant foods. Legumes, tofu, tempeh, seitan, nuts, seeds, and grains are excellent sources of protein, and when combined thoughtfully, they provide a wide spectrum of amino acids.

4. Supporting Muscle Health:

Protein plays a pivotal role in maintaining muscle health, making it vital for individuals engaged in physical activity or exercise. Whether one is a casual fitness enthusiast or a dedicated athlete, sufficient protein intake is necessary for muscle repair and growth.

5. Satiety and Weight Management:

Protein has been shown to enhance feelings of fullness and satiety. A diet rich in protein can help control appetite and reduce overall calorie consumption, which can be particularly beneficial for those looking to manage their weight.

6. Nutrient Absorption:

Protein also assists in the absorption of essential nutrients, including vitamins and minerals. It aids in transporting these vital compounds to cells throughout the body, ensuring that they are efficiently utilized.

7. Immune Function:

Proteins are integral to the immune system's function. Antibodies, which are proteins, are critical components of the body's defense against infections and diseases. Adequate protein intake supports a robust immune response.

8. Hair, Skin, and Nails:

Protein is a key component of hair, skin, and nails. Ensuring an adequate protein intake is essential for maintaining healthy and vibrant hair, clear skin, and strong nails.

9. Overall Health and Well-being:

A well-balanced vegan diet that includes an appropriate amount of protein is linked to numerous health benefits. It can help lower the risk of chronic diseases such as heart disease, type 2 diabetes, and certain cancers.

10. Achieving Optimal Nutrition:

To ensure optimal nutrition on a vegan diet, it's essential to focus not only on protein but also on other nutrients. Vegans should also pay attention to vitamin B12, iron, calcium, and omega-3 fatty acids, as these nutrients may require special attention in the absence of animal products.

Protein is an integral part of a vegan diet, as it supports various aspects of health, including muscle function, immune defense, and overall well-being. Vegans can easily meet their protein needs through a well-planned diet that incorporates a diverse range of plant-based protein sources. By embracing a balanced and protein-rich vegan lifestyle, individuals can enjoy the benefits of optimal nutrition while aligning their dietary choices with their ethical and environmental values.

Common Protein Sources for Vegans

Plant-based diets, which are gaining widespread popularity, offer an extensive range of protein sources essential for overall health. This is particularly relevant for vegans, vegetarians, and those looking to include more plant-based foods in their diets. Legumes, a key component of plant-based protein, offer variety and nutrition. Lentils, for example, are not only a protein powerhouse but also versatile, featuring in soups, stews, and salads. Chickpeas, the base for hummus, play a significant role in vegan dishes, particularly in Mediterranean and Middle Eastern cuisines. Black beans and kidney beans, staples in Latin American and various bean-based dishes, respectively, are perfect for an array of recipes like burritos, tacos, chili, and salads.

In the realm of soy-based products, tofu and tempeh stand out. Tofu, also known as bean curd, is incredibly adaptable and can be prepared in numerous ways including grilling, stir-frying, baking, and even blending into smoothies. Tempeh, a fermented product with a nutty flavor and firm texture, is excellent for sandwiches, stir-fries, and bowls. Seitan, or wheat gluten, known for its meaty texture, is another protein-rich option suitable for savory dishes.

Nuts and seeds, alongside their healthy fat content, are important protein sources. Almonds, peanuts, chia seeds, hemp seeds, and pumpkin seeds (pepitas) are nutritious and can be integrated into various meals and snacks. Whole grains such as quinoa, brown rice, and oats not only provide protein but also fiber, making them foundational in plant-based diets.

The rise of plant-based milk and yogurt alternatives has added to the variety. Variants like almond milk, soy milk, oat milk, and plant-based yogurts made from soy, almond, or coconut milk are often fortified with protein. Vegetables, sometimes overlooked, are also significant protein sources. Spinach, broccoli, Brussels sprouts, and peas are a few examples.

For those seeking meat alternatives, plant-based options such as veggie burgers, plant-based sausages, and meatless ground "beef" offer rich protein content. Legume-based pastas, made from chickpea or lentil flours, provide more protein than traditional wheat pasta. Additionally, vegan protein powders, often derived from pea, rice, or hemp proteins, can be an excellent addition to smoothies and recipes for a protein boost.

Incorporating these diverse plant-based protein sources into your diet ensures a wide range of delicious and nutritious meals, meeting protein requirements. A well-planned plant-based diet is capable of providing all essential nutrients for a balanced and healthy lifestyle. By thoughtfully planning meals and including a variety of these protein sources, vegans can easily meet their nutritional needs, enjoying a diverse and delightful range of plant-based meals. This approach not only aligns with ethical and environmental values but also ensures a well-rounded intake of essential nutrients.

Daily Protein Intake Recommendations

Protein is an essential nutrient that plays a vital role in various bodily functions, including tissue repair, immune support, and muscle maintenance. The daily protein intake recommendations can vary depending on factors such as age, gender, activity level, and overall health. Here are general guidelines for daily protein intake:

1. Recommended Dietary Allowance (RDA):

The Recommended Dietary Allowance (RDA) is the amount of protein that is considered sufficient to meet the nutritional needs of most healthy individuals. RDAs are established by health authorities to prevent deficiency and promote overall well-being.

- For adult men: The RDA for protein intake for adult men is approximately 56 grams per day.

- For adult women: The RDA for protein intake for adult women is approximately 46 grams per day.

It's important to note that these values are generalized and may not account for variations in individual needs based on factors like age, activity level, and health status.

2. Protein Needs Based on Activity Level:

Protein requirements can vary significantly based on physical activity levels. Individuals who engage in regular exercise, particularly strength training or endurance activities, may have higher protein needs to support muscle repair and growth.

- Sedentary individuals: Those who lead a sedentary lifestyle with minimal physical activity may find the RDA adequate.

- Active individuals: Those who engage in moderate physical activity or regular exercise may benefit from slightly higher protein intake, around 0.6 to 0.8 grams of protein per pound of body weight per day.

- Athletes: Competitive athletes or those with intense training regimens may require even more protein, ranging from 0.8 to 1.2 grams of protein per pound of body weight per day.

3. Protein Needs for Special Populations:

Certain populations have unique protein requirements:

- Pregnant and lactating women: Pregnant and breastfeeding women need additional protein to support fetal development and milk production. The recommended intake during pregnancy is approximately 71 grams per day, while lactating women may need around 71-75 grams per day.

- Infants and children: Protein needs are higher in growing children. Infants require around 10-15 grams of protein per day, while children and adolescents need protein based on their age, weight, and growth patterns.

- Older adults: Older adults may require slightly more protein to prevent muscle loss and maintain overall health. Aim for around 1.0 to 1.2 grams of protein per kilogram of body weight per day.

4. Individual Variations:

It's essential to recognize that individual protein needs can vary based on genetics, metabolism, and health conditions. Some medical conditions may necessitate higher or lower protein intake, and consulting with a healthcare professional or registered dietitian can provide personalized guidance.

5. Balanced Diet Considerations:

Incorporating a variety of protein sources into your diet, whether from plant-based or animal-based foods, can help ensure a well-rounded intake of essential amino acids and nutrients.

Remember that a balanced diet is key to overall health and well-being. It's important to consider not only the quantity of protein but also the quality and diversity of food sources to meet your daily protein intake recommendations while enjoying a variety of nutritious meals.

Factors Influencing Protein Needs

Protein is a fundamental macronutrient required for various bodily functions, including muscle maintenance, tissue repair, and the production of enzymes and hormones. However, individual protein needs can vary significantly based on several factors. Understanding these factors is essential for determining the appropriate protein intake for different individuals. Here are the key factors that influence protein needs:

1. Age:

- Protein needs tend to vary throughout the lifespan.

- Infants and children: Growing infants and children require more protein per unit of body weight to support rapid growth and development.

- Adults: Protein needs generally stabilize in adulthood but may increase slightly with aging to help maintain muscle mass and overall health.

- Older adults: Older adults may benefit from slightly higher protein intake to counteract age-related muscle loss and maintain optimal health.

2. Gender:

- Men often have slightly higher protein needs than women due to differences in muscle mass and overall body composition.

- However, individual variations in activity level and muscle mass can be more significant factors in determining protein needs than gender alone.

3. Activity Level:

- Physical activity and exercise can significantly impact protein requirements.

- Athletes and individuals engaged in regular strength training or endurance activities may have higher protein needs to support muscle repair and growth.

- Sedentary individuals typically require less protein than those with an active lifestyle.

4. Muscle Mass:

- Muscle mass plays a critical role in determining protein needs.

- Individuals with greater muscle mass may require more protein to support muscle maintenance and repair.

- Athletes, bodybuilders, and those aiming to build muscle may need higher protein intake.

5. Health Goals:

- Health and fitness goals can influence protein requirements.

- Weight loss: When aiming to lose weight, protein intake may need to be higher to help maintain muscle mass and promote satiety.

- Muscle gain: Individuals seeking to build muscle may require a protein-rich diet to support muscle protein synthesis.

- Recovery: Protein needs can increase during periods of injury, illness, or surgery to support tissue repair and healing.

6. Metabolism:

- Basal metabolic rate (BMR) and metabolism can affect daily protein needs.

- Faster metabolisms may require slightly more protein to support energy expenditure and maintain lean body mass.

- Slower metabolisms may require less protein.

7. Health Conditions:

- Certain health conditions can influence protein needs.

- Pregnancy and lactation: Pregnant and breastfeeding women require additional protein to support fetal development and milk production.

- Chronic illnesses or medical conditions: Some conditions may increase protein requirements, such as kidney disease, where protein intake may need to be restricted, or conditions that cause muscle wasting, where higher protein intake may be necessary.

8. Dietary Restrictions:

- Dietary choices, such as vegetarian or vegan diets, may require more careful planning to ensure adequate protein intake.

- Plant-based protein sources can provide sufficient protein when chosen wisely, but individuals may need to consume a variety of protein-rich plant foods to meet their needs.

9. Body Weight and Composition:

- Body weight, body composition, and overall energy expenditure can influence protein needs.

- Larger individuals and those with higher energy expenditure may require more protein to support their metabolic demands.

It's essential to recognize that individual protein needs are highly variable. To determine the appropriate protein intake for a specific person, it's advisable to consider these factors in combination and, when in doubt, consult with a healthcare professional or registered dietitian who can provide personalized guidance based on an individual's unique circumstances and goals.

Benefits of Whole Food Proteins

Benefits of whole food proteins extend beyond just their protein content; they offer a range of advantages for overall health and well-being.

Whole food proteins are often accompanied by a wealth of essential nutrients, including vitamins, minerals, fiber, and antioxidants. These nutrients play crucial roles in various bodily functions and contribute to overall vitality.

Furthermore, whole food proteins are typically minimally processed, preserving their natural nutritional integrity. Unlike heavily processed protein sources, whole foods are free from additives, preservatives, and excessive sodium, promoting better health outcomes.

Whole food proteins are often plant-based, which aligns with environmentally conscious and sustainable dietary choices. Plant-based proteins generally have a lower carbon footprint and require fewer resources to produce compared to animal-based proteins. This makes them a more eco-friendly option for those concerned about the environment.

Whole food proteins can be a boon for weight management. They tend to be rich in fiber, which enhances feelings of fullness and satiety, reducing overall calorie intake. This can be particularly beneficial for individuals looking to maintain or lose weight.

Moreover, whole food proteins are associated with improved heart health. They are typically low in saturated fats and cholesterol, reducing the risk of heart disease. Additionally, plant-based proteins may help lower blood pressure and cholesterol levels, contributing to cardiovascular well-being.

Lastly, whole food proteins offer diversity in dietary choices. Whether it's incorporating a variety of legumes, grains, nuts, or seeds, there are numerous options for creating delicious and nutritious meals. This variety not only keeps meals interesting but also ensures a wide range of nutrients are consumed.

In conclusion, whole food proteins are a valuable component of a balanced diet, offering an array of benefits ranging from nutritional richness and sustainability to heart health and weight management. By embracing whole food protein sources, individuals can support their overall health while making environmentally responsible food choices.

Balancing Macronutrients in a Vegan Diet

A well-balanced diet is essential for optimal health, and this holds true for vegan diets as well. Balancing macronutrients—carbohydrates, proteins, and fats—in a vegan diet is crucial to ensure that you receive the necessary nutrients for energy, growth, and overall well-being. Here's how to balance macronutrients effectively in a vegan diet:

1. Carbohydrates:

Carbohydrates are a primary source of energy and should constitute a significant portion of your daily calorie intake. Focus on complex carbohydrates from whole, unprocessed foods, such as:

- Whole grains: Incorporate foods like brown rice, quinoa, oats, whole wheat bread, and whole wheat pasta into your meals. These provide sustained energy and essential nutrients.

- Legumes: Lentils, chickpeas, black beans, and other legumes are rich in carbohydrates, fiber, and protein, making them excellent additions to a vegan diet.

- Fruits and vegetables: These provide essential vitamins, minerals, and fiber. Aim for a colorful variety to maximize nutrient intake.

2. Protein:

Protein is essential for muscle maintenance, tissue repair, and overall health. As a vegan, you can obtain ample protein from plant-based sources, such as:

- Legumes: Beans, lentils, chickpeas, and peas are excellent sources of plant-based protein.

- Tofu and tempeh: These soy-based products are rich in protein and can be incorporated into a variety of dishes.

- Nuts and seeds: Almonds, peanuts, chia seeds, and hemp seeds contain protein and healthy fats.

- Whole grains: Quinoa, farro, and bulgur also provide protein in addition to carbohydrates.

Ensure that you include a variety of protein sources in your meals to obtain a wide range of essential amino acids. Combining different plant-based proteins, such as beans and rice or tofu and quinoa, can help achieve a complete amino acid profile.

3. Fats:

Fats are essential for overall health, including hormone production and absorption of fat-soluble vitamins. Choose healthy sources of fats in a vegan diet, such as:

- Avocados: Rich in monounsaturated fats and fiber, avocados provide a creamy texture to dishes.

- Nuts and seeds: These are good sources of healthy fats, but consume them in moderation due to their calorie density.

- Oils: Use plant-based oils like olive oil, coconut oil, and avocado oil for cooking and salad dressings.

- Nut butters: Natural nut and seed butters, like almond butter and tahini, are rich in healthy fats.

4. Fiber:

Fiber is essential for digestive health and helps maintain stable blood sugar levels. Vegan diets are naturally high in fiber due to the abundance of plant-based foods. Ensure you consume a variety of fruits, vegetables, whole grains, and legumes to maximize your fiber intake.

5. Micronutrients:

Pay attention to micronutrients such as vitamins and minerals. Vegan diets can be rich in certain nutrients like folate, vitamin C, and antioxidants found in plant-based foods. However, be mindful of nutrients like vitamin B12, iron, calcium, and omega-3 fatty acids, which may require special attention or supplementation in a vegan diet.

A balanced vegan diet involves incorporating a variety of whole, plant-based foods to provide a well-rounded intake of macronutrients, micronutrients, and fiber. By planning meals thoughtfully and paying attention to nutrient-rich sources, vegans can enjoy a healthy and nutritionally complete diet that aligns with ethical and environmental values.

Cooking with Plant Proteins

Cooking with plant proteins opens up a world of culinary possibilities while promoting health and sustainability. Plant-based proteins are versatile, offering a wide range of textures and flavors that can be incorporated into various dishes. Whether you're a dedicated vegan or simply looking to reduce your meat consumption, here are some exciting ways to get creative with plant proteins in the kitchen.

One popular plant protein source is tofu, known for its ability to absorb flavors and adapt to various cooking methods. Tofu can be cubed, sliced, or crumbled to create a variety of textures. It's perfect for stir-fries, marinating in savory sauces, grilling, or blending into creamy smoothies and desserts. Silken tofu is a fantastic base for vegan cheesecakes and creamy salad dressings.

Another beloved plant protein is tempeh, which boasts a nutty flavor and firm texture. Tempeh is ideal for marinating and grilling, making it a great substitute for meat in sandwiches and burgers. It can also be crumbled and used as a protein-rich topping for salads or tacos.

Lentils and legumes are excellent additions to plant-based meals, offering protein and fiber. Red lentils are perfect for thickening soups and creating creamy, protein-packed dals. Chickpeas, when mashed and seasoned, can be transformed into tasty falafel or chickpea burgers. Beans, such as black beans or kidney beans, can be used in chili, stews, and even brownies for added moisture and protein.

Quinoa, often referred to as a "complete protein," is a versatile grain that can be used in place of rice or couscous in various dishes. It's a valuable addition to salads, grain bowls, or stuffed bell peppers. Quinoa also makes a nutritious base for breakfast bowls topped with fruits and nuts.

Nuts and seeds, like almonds, cashews, chia seeds, and hemp seeds, are packed with protein and healthy fats. They can be ground into nut butters, sprinkled on salads, or used as toppings for oatmeal and yogurt. Nut butters, in particular, can be blended into savory sauces, dressings, and desserts, offering a creamy texture and a rich, nutty flavor.

Plant-based protein powders, made from sources like pea, rice, or hemp protein, are convenient options for boosting the protein content of smoothies, pancakes, or baked goods. These powders are available in various flavors, allowing you to experiment with different taste profiles.

Cooking with plant proteins isn't limited to just replicating meat-based dishes; it's an opportunity to explore diverse cuisines and flavors. Asian-inspired stir-fries with tofu and vegetables, hearty Italian pasta dishes with lentil-based sauces, and Mexican tacos with spiced black bean filling are just a few examples of the culinary delights that plant proteins can offer. Whether you're an experienced cook or new to plant-based cooking, there are endless possibilities to explore and enjoy while reaping the health and environmental benefits of plant-based proteins.

Why Consider Protein Supplements?

Protein supplements have become increasingly popular among individuals pursuing various health and fitness goals. While obtaining protein from whole foods is generally recommended, there are several reasons why someone might consider protein supplements as part of their dietary regimen.

One primary reason is convenience. Protein supplements are quick and easy to prepare, making them a convenient option for people with busy lifestyles. Whether it's a protein shake, bar, or powder, these products can provide a readily available source of protein, especially when time is limited.

Athletes and fitness enthusiasts often turn to protein supplements to support muscle recovery and growth. After intense exercise, the body's demand for protein increases. Protein supplements can help deliver amino acids to muscles more rapidly, aiding in the repair and rebuilding of muscle tissue.

For those following specific dietary patterns, such as vegans or vegetarians, protein supplements can be a valuable tool. It can sometimes be challenging to meet protein needs solely through plant-based sources, and protein supplements can help bridge the gap, ensuring adequate protein intake.

Individuals aiming for weight management or weight loss may also find protein supplements beneficial. Protein has a satiating effect, helping to reduce feelings of hunger and promote fullness. By incorporating protein supplements into their diet, people can better control their calorie intake and support their weight loss efforts.

In some cases, medical conditions or surgeries may require higher protein intake for healing and recovery. Protein supplements can provide an easily digestible and concentrated source of protein to meet these increased needs during times of illness or post-surgery recuperation.

Protein supplements are not only used for sports and fitness purposes but also as a convenient option for elderly individuals or those with reduced appetite who may struggle to consume adequate protein through regular meals. In such cases, protein supplements can help maintain muscle mass and overall health.

It's important to note that while protein supplements can be beneficial in specific situations, they should not replace whole food sources of protein in a balanced diet. Whole foods offer a broader range of essential nutrients, fiber, and phytochemicals that contribute to overall health.

Ultimately, the decision to consider protein supplements should be based on individual goals, lifestyle, and dietary preferences. Consulting with a healthcare professional or registered dietitian can provide personalized guidance on whether protein supplements are appropriate and how to incorporate them effectively into a dietary plan.

Types of Protein Supplements for Vegans

Vegans have a variety of protein supplements to choose from to meet their dietary needs and fitness goals. These supplements offer convenient and concentrated sources of plant-based protein, ensuring that vegans can maintain an adequate protein intake without relying solely on whole foods.

One of the most common types of protein supplements for vegans is plant-based protein powders. These powders are typically derived from sources like pea protein, rice protein, hemp protein, or a blend of these plant sources. They are highly versatile and can be easily incorporated into smoothies, oatmeal, baking recipes, and more. Plant-based protein powders are known for their rich amino acid profiles, making them a suitable option for those seeking to build and repair muscle.

Soy protein isolate is another popular vegan protein supplement. It's derived from soybeans and contains all the essential amino acids, making it a complete protein source. Soy protein isolate is available in various forms, including powders, bars, and ready-to-drink shakes. It's known for its smooth texture and neutral flavor, making it suitable for a wide range of recipes and applications.

For individuals with specific dietary preferences or allergies, pea protein has gained popularity. Pea protein isolate is often used in plant-based protein supplements due to its high protein content and digestibility. It's particularly appealing to those who may have soy or gluten allergies. Pea protein supplements are available in various flavors and can be a convenient choice for vegans looking to meet their protein needs.

Hemp protein is derived from hemp seeds and is known for its high fiber content in addition to protein. While it may not have as high a protein concentration as other sources, it offers additional nutritional benefits, including essential fatty acids and minerals. Hemp protein supplements can be added to smoothies, yogurt, or used in baking for an extra nutrient boost.

Nutritional protein bars are another convenient option for vegans on the go. These bars often contain a combination of plant-based protein sources, along with other ingredients like nuts, seeds, and dried fruits. They provide a quick and portable way to increase protein intake between meals or as a post-workout snack.

Fortified plant-based milks and yogurts are becoming increasingly popular as protein sources. Some brands add additional protein to their dairy alternatives by fortifying them with ingredients like pea protein or almond protein. These products offer a tasty and convenient way to boost protein intake while enjoying the creamy texture of traditional dairy products.

It's important to note that when selecting protein supplements, it's essential to read labels carefully to ensure they align with your dietary preferences and goals. Look for products with minimal additives and artificial ingredients. Additionally, consulting with a registered dietitian can provide personalized guidance on choosing the right protein supplements and incorporating them effectively into your vegan diet to meet your nutritional needs.

Pea Protein Isolate: A Plant-Powered Protein Option

Pea protein isolate has gained popularity as a plant-based protein source in recent years, and for good reason. Derived from yellow split peas, this protein supplement offers a range of benefits that make it an attractive option for vegans, vegetarians, and individuals with dietary restrictions or preferences.

One of the key advantages of pea protein isolate is its impressive protein content. It typically contains about 85-90% protein by weight, making it a concentrated source of amino acids. This high protein concentration makes it suitable for those looking to meet their protein needs for muscle building, recovery, or weight management.

Another notable benefit of pea protein isolate is its suitability for individuals with common food allergies and sensitivities. It is naturally free from major allergens like dairy, gluten, and soy, making it an excellent choice for those with lactose intolerance, celiac disease, or soy allergies. Additionally, pea protein is easy to digest and less likely to cause digestive discomfort compared to some other protein sources.

Pea protein isolate has a well-balanced amino acid profile, although it may be slightly lower in one amino acid, methionine, compared to animal-based proteins. To ensure a complete amino acid intake, it's recommended to combine pea protein with other plant-based protein sources, such as rice protein or hemp protein. This combination creates a complete protein profile that supports muscle maintenance and overall health.

For those concerned about sustainability and environmental impact, pea protein is a more eco-friendly choice compared to some animal-based proteins. Peas are a nitrogen-fixing crop, which means they can enrich the soil with nitrogen, reducing the need for synthetic fertilizers. Additionally, growing peas typically requires less water and produces fewer greenhouse gas emissions compared to animal agriculture.

Pea protein isolate is versatile and can be used in a variety of recipes and applications. It has a mild, neutral flavor that blends well in smoothies, shakes, and baked goods. Many brands offer flavored pea protein powders, including chocolate, vanilla, and unflavored options, catering to different taste preferences.

While pea protein isolate offers numerous benefits, it's essential to read labels carefully when selecting a product. Some pea protein supplements may contain added sugars, artificial flavors, or fillers. Choose products with minimal additives and opt for those that have undergone third-party testing for quality and safety.

Rice Protein: A Plant-Based Protein Alternative

Rice protein is a plant-based protein option that has gained popularity among individuals seeking alternative protein sources, especially those following vegan or vegetarian diets. Derived from brown or white rice, this protein supplement offers a range of benefits and applications.

One of the primary advantages of rice protein is its hypoallergenic nature. It is naturally free from common allergens such as dairy, gluten, and soy, making it an excellent choice for individuals with food allergies or sensitivities. This hypoallergenic quality ensures that rice protein is gentle on the digestive system and less likely to cause allergic reactions.

Rice protein isolate, in particular, boasts a high protein content, typically around 80-90% protein by weight. This concentration makes it an attractive option for those looking to increase their protein intake, whether for muscle building, weight management, or overall health. It provides a rich source of essential amino acids, including all nine that the body cannot produce on its own.

While rice protein is a valuable plant-based protein source, it may be slightly lower in one specific amino acid, lysine, compared to animal-based proteins. To ensure a well-rounded amino acid profile, individuals can combine rice protein with other plant-based proteins, such as pea protein or hemp protein, to create a complete protein source that supports muscle maintenance and overall nutrition.

Rice protein is easy to digest and has a mild, neutral flavor, making it suitable for a wide range of recipes and applications. It can be added to smoothies, shakes, oatmeal, or used in baking to boost the protein content of various dishes. Some flavored rice protein powders are available on the market, catering to different taste preferences.

Additionally, rice protein is often considered a sustainable choice. Rice cultivation typically requires less water compared to some other crops, and rice protein production can have a lower environmental impact when compared to animal agriculture. Choosing rice protein can align with eco-conscious dietary choices.

When selecting a rice protein product, it's important to read labels carefully. Some rice protein supplements may contain additives, sweeteners, or fillers. Opt for products with minimal additives and choose those that have undergone third-party testing for quality and safety.

Hemp Protein: A Nutrient-Rich Plant-Based Protein

Hemp protein is derived from hemp seeds and has gained recognition as a nutritious plant-based protein source. Hemp has been cultivated for thousands of years for its versatile uses, including as a protein-rich dietary staple. Today, hemp protein offers numerous health benefits and culinary applications.

One of the standout qualities of hemp protein is its impressive nutrient profile. It is a complete protein source, meaning it contains all nine essential amino acids that the body cannot produce on its own. This makes hemp protein a valuable option for individuals looking to support muscle maintenance and overall health.

Hemp protein is not only rich in protein but also packed with essential fatty acids, particularly omega-3 and omega-6 fatty acids. These fats play a crucial role in heart health, brain function, and inflammation regulation. Hemp protein can be a valuable addition to a balanced diet, especially for those seeking to increase their intake of these beneficial fats.

Additionally, hemp protein is a good source of dietary fiber, which aids in digestion and promotes feelings of fullness and satiety. The fiber content can support healthy digestion and may contribute to weight management goals.

Hemp protein is often well-tolerated by individuals with dietary restrictions or allergies. It is naturally gluten-free and dairy-free, making it suitable for those with celiac disease, lactose intolerance, or soy allergies. Its hypoallergenic nature ensures that it is gentle on the digestive system and less likely to cause discomfort.

The flavor of hemp protein is typically described as nutty and earthy, which can add depth to various dishes. It can be blended into smoothies, stirred into yogurt, incorporated into baking recipes, or sprinkled over salads for a protein boost. Some flavored hemp protein powders are available, catering to different taste preferences.

From an environmental perspective, hemp is considered a sustainable crop. It grows quickly and requires minimal pesticides and water, making it a more eco-friendly option compared to some other agricultural practices.

Choosing hemp protein aligns with environmentally conscious dietary choices.

When selecting a hemp protein product, ensure it is derived from reputable sources that prioritize quality and safety. Look for products that have undergone third-party testing to confirm their purity and nutrient content.

Soy Protein: A Versatile Plant-Based Protein

Soy protein is one of the most well-established and widely recognized plant-based protein sources available. Derived from soybeans, it has been a dietary staple in various cultures for centuries and is known for its versatility and numerous health benefits.

One of the key advantages of soy protein is its exceptional protein content. It is considered a complete protein source, containing all nine essential amino acids that the body cannot produce on its own. This makes soy protein an excellent choice for individuals seeking to meet their protein needs, whether for muscle building, recovery, or overall health.

Soy protein isolate, a highly concentrated form of soy protein, is particularly popular among athletes and fitness enthusiasts. It boasts a protein content of approximately 90% by weight, providing a potent source of amino acids. This concentration makes it suitable for those looking to increase their protein intake without consuming excess calories.

Beyond protein, soy protein offers additional health benefits. It is known for its potential to support heart health by reducing LDL (bad) cholesterol levels. This heart-healthy attribute is attributed to bioactive compounds called isoflavones, which can help improve blood lipid profiles.

Soy protein is also rich in other nutrients, including iron, calcium, and various B vitamins. These nutrients are essential for overall health and well-being and make soy protein a valuable addition to a balanced diet.

One of the notable qualities of soy protein is its versatility. It can be incorporated into a wide range of recipes and applications, from savory dishes like tofu stir-fries and soy-based meat alternatives to sweet treats like soy milk and soy-based desserts. Soy protein's neutral flavor allows it to take on various tastes and textures, making it a suitable ingredient for both savory and sweet dishes.

While soy protein is highly regarded for its nutritional benefits, it's essential to consider individual dietary preferences and potential allergens. Some individuals may have soy allergies or prefer to limit soy intake due to concerns about phytoestrogens, naturally occurring compounds in soy. In such cases, there are alternative plant-based protein sources like pea protein, rice protein, or hemp protein that can be considered.

When selecting soy protein products, it's advisable to choose those from reputable sources that prioritize quality and safety. Opt for non-GMO (genetically modified organism) and organic soy protein options if you have specific preferences.

In conclusion, soy protein is a versatile and nutrient-rich plant-based protein source with numerous health benefits. Whether you follow a vegan or vegetarian diet, are concerned about heart health, or simply want to incorporate a valuable protein source into your meals, soy protein can be an excellent addition to your dietary plan.

Brown Rice Protein: A Plant-Based Protein with a Nutritional Punch

Brown rice protein is a plant-based protein source that has gained popularity among individuals seeking alternative protein options, particularly those following vegan or vegetarian diets. Derived from whole brown rice grains, this protein supplement offers several health benefits and culinary versatility.

One of the primary advantages of brown rice protein is its natural origin. Unlike many protein isolates, it is minimally processed, typically made by simply removing the carbohydrates and fiber from brown rice grains. This minimal processing helps retain the nutritional integrity of the rice, ensuring that essential nutrients like vitamins, minerals, and antioxidants are preserved.

Brown rice protein is rich in protein, with a protein content that varies between 70% to 80% by weight, depending on the product. This concentration makes it a valuable option for those looking to increase their protein intake, whether for muscle building, recovery, or overall health. It provides essential amino acids, including all nine that the body cannot produce on its own.

For individuals with dietary restrictions or allergies, brown rice protein is a suitable choice. It is naturally free from common allergens like dairy, gluten, and soy, making it an excellent option for those with specific dietary needs. Its hypoallergenic properties ensure that it is gentle on the digestive system and less likely to cause discomfort.

Brown rice protein is known for its mild and neutral flavor, which makes it adaptable for various culinary applications. It can be incorporated into smoothies, shakes, oatmeal, or used in baking recipes to boost the protein content of a wide range of dishes. Some flavored brown rice protein powders are available on the market, catering to different taste preferences.

From an environmental perspective, brown rice cultivation is considered a sustainable choice. It typically requires less water compared to some other crops, contributing to more efficient water usage in agriculture. Choosing brown rice protein aligns with eco-conscious dietary choices.

When selecting a brown rice protein product, it's essential to read labels carefully. Some brown rice protein supplements may contain additives, sweeteners, or fillers. Opt for products with minimal additives and choose those that have undergone third-party testing for quality and safety.

Pumpkin Seed Protein: A Nutrient-Packed Plant-Based Protein

Pumpkin seed protein is a lesser-known but highly nutritious plant-based protein source that offers a range of health benefits. Derived from pumpkin seeds, this protein supplement is gaining recognition for its nutrient density and versatility.

One of the standout qualities of pumpkin seed protein is its impressive protein content. It typically contains around 60-70% protein by weight, making it a concentrated source of amino acids. While it may not have the highest protein content compared to some other protein sources, it offers additional nutritional advantages.

Pumpkin seed protein is a complete protein source, meaning it provides all nine essential amino acids that the body cannot produce on its own. This makes it suitable for individuals seeking to support muscle maintenance, recovery, and overall health.

Beyond protein, pumpkin seed protein is packed with essential nutrients. It is particularly rich in minerals like magnesium, zinc, and iron. Magnesium supports muscle and nerve function, zinc is essential for immune health, and iron helps transport oxygen in the blood. These minerals contribute to the overall nutritional value of pumpkin seed protein.

Pumpkin seed protein is also a good source of dietary fiber, which aids in digestion and promotes feelings of fullness and satiety. The fiber content can support healthy digestion and may contribute to weight management goals.

The flavor of pumpkin seed protein is typically described as nutty and earthy, which can add depth to various dishes. It can be blended into smoothies, stirred into yogurt, incorporated into baking recipes, or sprinkled over salads for a protein boost.

Pumpkin seed protein is well-tolerated by most individuals and is naturally free from common allergens like dairy, gluten, and soy. This makes it a suitable choice for those with dietary restrictions or allergies.

From an environmental perspective, pumpkin seeds are a sustainable crop. They require relatively low water usage compared to some other agricultural practices, contributing to more efficient water conservation. Choosing pumpkin seed protein aligns with eco-conscious dietary choices.

When selecting a pumpkin seed protein product, it's essential to read labels carefully. Some products may contain additives, sweeteners, or fillers. Opt for products with minimal additives and choose those that have undergone third-party testing for quality and safety.

Sunflower Seed Protein: A Nutrient-Rich Plant-Based Option

Sunflower seed protein is an emerging plant-based protein source that offers numerous health benefits and culinary possibilities. Derived from sunflower seeds, this protein supplement is gaining recognition for its nutrient density and versatility.

One of the key advantages of sunflower seed protein is its impressive protein content. It typically contains around 45-50% protein by weight, making it a concentrated source of amino acids. While it may not have the highest protein content compared to some other protein sources, it offers additional nutritional advantages.

Sunflower seed protein is considered a complete protein source, providing all nine essential amino acids that the body cannot produce on its own. This makes it suitable for individuals looking to support muscle maintenance, recovery, and overall health.

In addition to protein, sunflower seed protein is rich in essential nutrients. It is notably high in vitamins and minerals, including vitamin E, magnesium, and selenium. Vitamin E is an antioxidant that helps protect cells from oxidative damage, while magnesium supports muscle and nerve function, and selenium contributes to overall health.

Sunflower seed protein is also a good source of dietary fiber, which aids in digestion and promotes feelings of fullness and satiety. The fiber content can support healthy digestion and may contribute to weight management goals.

The flavor of sunflower seed protein is generally mild and nutty, making it versatile for various culinary applications. It can be blended into smoothies, stirred into yogurt, incorporated into baking recipes, or sprinkled over salads for a protein boost.

Sunflower seed protein is naturally free from common allergens like dairy, gluten, and soy, making it suitable for individuals with dietary restrictions or allergies. It is generally well-tolerated by most individuals and is easy on the digestive system.

From an environmental perspective, sunflower cultivation is considered relatively sustainable. Sunflowers are known for their ability to grow in diverse climates and require less water compared to some other crops. Choosing sunflower seed protein aligns with eco-conscious dietary choices.

When selecting a sunflower seed protein product, it's essential to read labels carefully. Some products may contain additives, sweeteners, or fillers. Opt for products with minimal additives and choose those that have undergone third-party testing for quality and safety.

Combination Blends: Maximizing the Benefits of Plant-Based Proteins

Combination blends of plant-based proteins have gained popularity as a way to maximize the nutritional benefits and culinary versatility of these protein sources. These blends typically consist of two or more plant-based protein types, each with its unique amino acid profile and nutritional advantages.

One of the primary advantages of combination blends is their ability to provide a more complete and balanced amino acid profile. Different plant-based proteins may be slightly deficient in specific essential amino acids, but when combined, they complement each other, creating a well-rounded source of protein. This is particularly important for individuals seeking to support muscle building, recovery, and overall health.

Common combinations include blends of pea protein, rice protein, and hemp protein. Pea protein is rich in lysine but lower in methionine, while rice protein has the opposite profile. Hemp protein adds extra nutrients like essential fatty acids and fiber to the mix. These combinations ensure that the essential amino acid needs of the body are met.

Combination blends also offer a broader range of vitamins and minerals. Different plant-based proteins may naturally contain varying levels of essential nutrients. By blending various protein sources, individuals can benefit from a more diverse nutrient profile, which contributes to overall health and well-being.

From a culinary perspective, combination blends provide a flexible and versatile ingredient for a wide range of recipes. The neutral flavors of some protein sources make them adaptable for both sweet and savory dishes. Blends can be added to smoothies, baked goods, soups, and more to increase the protein content and nutritional value of meals.

Combination blends are suitable for individuals with dietary restrictions or allergies since they often consist of allergen-free protein sources. This inclusivity makes them a valuable option for those with specific dietary needs.

When selecting a combination blend, it's important to choose products from reputable sources that prioritize quality and safety. Read labels carefully to ensure that the blend aligns with your dietary preferences and goals. Look for blends that have undergone third-party testing to verify their purity and nutrient content.

Protein Powder Selection Guide

Selecting the right protein powder can be a crucial decision, as it plays a significant role in your dietary and fitness goals. Whether you're looking for a protein powder for muscle building, weight management, or overall health, consider this protein powder selection guide to make an informed choice:

1. Protein Source:

- Choose a protein source that aligns with your dietary preferences and any allergies or sensitivities. Common options include whey protein (for dairy consumers), plant-based proteins (such as pea, rice, hemp, or soy), and collagen protein.

2. Protein Concentration:

- Protein powders come in various concentrations, ranging from 50% to 90% protein by weight. If your goal is to increase protein intake without many additional calories, opt for a higher protein concentration. For added nutrients, choose a lower concentration with more fats and carbs.

3. Dietary Goals:

- Consider your dietary goals when selecting a protein powder. If you're looking to build muscle, a protein powder with a rich amino acid profile and high protein content is ideal. For weight management, opt for a lower-calorie protein powder with minimal added sugars and fats.

4. Allergen-Free Options:

- If you have food allergies or intolerances, check for allergen-free protein powders that are free from common allergens like dairy, gluten, and soy.

5. Flavors and Additives:

- Protein powders come in various flavors, from chocolate and vanilla to exotic options. Be mindful of added sugars and artificial sweeteners. Opt for products with minimal additives, fillers, or artificial ingredients.

6. Sweeteners:

- Some protein powders are sweetened with natural sweeteners like stevia or monk fruit, while others may contain sugar alcohols or artificial sweeteners. Choose a protein powder with sweeteners that align with your preferences and dietary restrictions.

7. Texture and Mixability:

- Consider the texture and mixability of the protein powder. Some protein powders blend well with water or milk, while others may clump or have a gritty texture. Read reviews and user feedback for insights into mixability.

8. Purpose:

- Different protein powders may be designed for specific purposes. For example, whey protein isolate is often favored for post-workout recovery, while casein protein is known for its slow digestion and suitability as a nighttime snack.

9. Brand Reputation:

- Research the brand's reputation, certifications, and third-party testing for quality and safety. Look for products from reputable companies that prioritize transparency and quality control.

10. Price and Value:

- Compare prices per serving and serving sizes to assess the overall value of the protein powder. Consider whether the product aligns with your budget and provides the protein content you need.

11. Personal Taste:

- Ultimately, personal taste matters. Experiment with different protein powders to find one that suits your taste buds and preferences. Many brands offer sample sizes for you to try before committing to a larger container.

Remember that protein supplements should complement a balanced diet, and whole food sources of protein should remain a significant part of your nutrition. Consult with a healthcare professional or registered dietitian for personalized guidance based on your specific dietary goals and needs when selecting a protein powder that's right for you.

Understanding Nutritional Labels: Making Informed Dietary Choices

Nutritional labels are an essential tool for making informed dietary choices and understanding the nutritional content of food products. These labels provide valuable information about the composition, serving size, and nutrient content of the food item, helping consumers make healthier decisions.

One of the key elements of a nutritional label is the serving size. This represents the amount of food or drink considered as one serving and serves as a reference point for the other nutrition information on the label. Paying attention to the serving size is crucial, as it affects the accuracy of nutrient values. It's essential to compare the serving size to the amount you intend to consume to get an accurate understanding of the nutrients you'll be consuming.

Calories are another important component of nutritional labels. They represent the energy content of one serving of the food. Understanding the calorie content can help you manage your daily calorie intake, especially if you're working towards weight management goals.

Nutritional labels also provide information about macronutrients, which include carbohydrates, proteins, and fats. Carbohydrates are further broken down into dietary fiber and sugars. Proteins and fats are usually presented as total amounts per serving. Monitoring these macronutrients can help individuals balance their diet according to their nutritional needs.

Dietary fiber is a valuable component to consider, as it supports digestive health and can contribute to feelings of fullness and satiety. Pay attention to the amount of dietary fiber in a product, especially if you're aiming to increase your fiber intake.

Sugars, on the other hand, should be monitored, as excessive sugar consumption can contribute to various health issues. Differentiate between natural sugars, such as those found in fruits, and added sugars, which are incorporated during food processing.

Fats on the label can be further broken down into different types of fats, including saturated fats and trans fats. Limiting the intake of saturated and trans fats is advisable, as they are associated with an increased risk of heart disease. Instead, focus on unsaturated fats, which are healthier options.

Nutritional labels also provide information on essential vitamins and minerals, such as vitamin D, calcium, iron, and potassium. Understanding these values can help ensure you're meeting your daily nutrient requirements.

Percent Daily Value (DV) is another feature on nutritional labels. It indicates how much one serving of the food contributes to your daily nutrient needs based on a 2,000-calorie diet. Keep in mind that individual nutrient requirements may vary, so the DV may not align with your specific needs.

When interpreting nutritional labels, it's essential to consider your dietary goals and any dietary restrictions or preferences you may have. Reading labels can help you make informed choices that align with your nutritional needs and health objectives.

Certifications and Quality Standards: Ensuring the Safety and Integrity of Food Products

Certifications and quality standards play a crucial role in ensuring the safety, authenticity, and quality of food products in the marketplace. These certifications are a testament to a product's adherence to specific criteria, which can vary widely depending on the type of certification and the organization responsible for it.

One of the most well-known certifications is the USDA Organic certification. This certification ensures that food products meet strict organic farming and processing standards. Organic foods are grown without synthetic pesticides, herbicides, or genetically modified organisms (GMOs). They also adhere to certain animal welfare and sustainability guidelines. Consumers who prioritize organic products can look for the USDA Organic seal on labels to make informed choices.

Another significant certification is the Non-GMO Project Verified seal. This certification indicates that a product does not contain genetically modified organisms. It provides consumers with the assurance that the product's ingredients have been tested and verified to be non-GMO. As concerns about GMOs and their potential health and environmental impacts continue to grow, this certification has become increasingly important.

Fair Trade certification is another notable standard that focuses on ethical and sustainable sourcing practices. Fair Trade ensures that farmers and workers in developing countries receive fair wages and have safe working conditions. This certification extends to various products, including coffee, cocoa, and certain fruits. It allows consumers to support ethical trade practices and sustainability while enjoying their favorite products.

For individuals with dietary restrictions or allergies, certifications like Gluten-Free, Kosher, and Halal are essential. These certifications help consumers identify products that meet specific dietary requirements. Gluten-Free certification is especially crucial for individuals with celiac disease or gluten sensitivities, ensuring that products are safe to consume.

Animal welfare certifications, such as Certified Humane or Animal Welfare Approved, focus on the treatment of animals in food production. These certifications guarantee that animals are raised under humane conditions, with access to open spaces, clean environments, and proper care. Ethical treatment of animals is a priority for many consumers, and these certifications allow them to support these practices.

Sustainability certifications, like the Marine Stewardship Council (MSC) label for seafood or Rainforest Alliance for various products, signal that products are sourced and produced in environmentally responsible ways. They ensure that fisheries and farms adhere to sustainable practices that protect ecosystems and support long-term environmental health.

When consumers see these certifications on food labels, they can have confidence that the product meets specific standards aligned with their values and dietary needs. It's essential to educate oneself about the various certifications and what they represent to make informed choices that support personal health, ethical values, and environmental sustainability.

Avoiding Common Additives and Allergens: Navigating Food Labels for Health and Safety

Food labels provide crucial information about the ingredients used in a product, including common additives and potential allergens. Understanding how to read labels and identify these elements is essential for individuals who want to make informed choices to protect their health and safety.

Common Additives:

Many packaged foods contain additives to enhance flavor, extend shelf life, or improve texture. Some additives are considered safe for consumption, while others may raise concerns for some individuals. It's important to be aware of additives and their potential effects. For instance, some people may wish to avoid artificial food colorings or preservatives like sodium benzoate due to concerns about hyperactivity or sensitivity.

Reading the ingredient list on food labels is the most effective way to identify common additives. Look for names of additives you want to avoid, and be cautious of terms like "artificial flavors" or "artificial sweeteners," as they may indicate the presence of additives.

Allergens:

Food allergies can trigger severe reactions, making it crucial to identify potential allergens in packaged foods. Common allergens include peanuts, tree nuts, milk, eggs, soy, wheat, fish, and shellfish. Food labels in many countries are required to clearly list these allergens in the ingredient list or with a separate allergen statement.

For individuals with food allergies, it's essential to read labels carefully and identify any allergens mentioned. Cross-contamination is another concern, as allergens can unintentionally find their way into other products during manufacturing processes. Look for precautionary statements like "may contain traces of..." or "processed in a facility that also handles..." to assess the risk of cross-contamination.

Gluten and Gluten-Free Labeling:

Gluten is a protein found in wheat, barley, rye, and their derivatives. For individuals with celiac disease or gluten sensitivity, avoiding gluten is crucial. Gluten-free labeling helps these individuals identify safe products. In many countries, gluten-free labeling is regulated and requires products labeled as such to meet specific gluten content criteria.

Reading Labels:

To navigate food labels effectively, start by reading the ingredient list carefully. The most critical information is typically found near the beginning of the list, as ingredients are listed in descending order of quantity. If you need to avoid a particular additive or allergen, ensure it's not listed in the ingredient list.

Pay attention to allergen statements and precautionary labels about cross-contamination. These can provide insights into the safety of the product for individuals with allergies.

Understanding food labels empowers consumers to make choices that align with their dietary needs and health goals. Whether you're avoiding common additives, allergens, or gluten, thorough label reading is essential for ensuring your health and safety when selecting packaged foods.

High Protein Vegan Smoothie Recipes

1. Vegan Green Protein Smoothie

Ingredients:

- 1 cup of unsweetened almond milk (or any plant-based milk)

- 1 scoop of vegan protein powder (pea protein or hemp protein works well)

- 1 cup of fresh spinach leaves

- 1/2 frozen banana

- 1 tablespoon of almond butter

- 1 tablespoon of chia seeds

- 1/2 teaspoon of cinnamon

- Ice cubes (optional)

- Sweetener (such as agave nectar or dates) to taste

Instructions:

Place almond milk, vegan protein powder, spinach, frozen banana, almond butter, chia seeds, and cinnamon in a blender.

Blend until all ingredients are thoroughly combined and the smoothie is creamy.

If you want it colder, add some ice cubes and blend again.

Taste and sweeten with agave nectar or pitted dates if desired.

Pour into a glass and enjoy your protein-packed green smoothie!

2. Vegan Berry Protein Powerhouse Smoothie

Ingredients:

- 1 cup of mixed berries (strawberries, blueberries, raspberries)

- 1 cup of silken tofu (for added creaminess and protein)

- 1 scoop of vegan protein powder (rice protein or soy protein)

- 1 tablespoon of flaxseeds

- 1 cup of unsweetened almond milk (or any plant-based milk)

- Ice cubes (optional)

- Sweetener (such as maple syrup or agave nectar) to taste

Instructions:

Combine mixed berries, silken tofu, vegan protein powder, flaxseeds, and almond milk in a blender.

Blend until all ingredients are well combined and the smoothie is smooth.

Add ice cubes if you want a colder smoothie and blend briefly.

Sweeten with maple syrup or agave nectar if needed.

Pour into a glass and enjoy this berry-packed protein powerhouse!

3. Vegan Chocolate Peanut Butter Protein Shake

Ingredients:

- 1 cup of unsweetened chocolate almond milk (or any plant-based chocolate milk)

- 1 scoop of vegan chocolate protein powder

- 2 tablespoons of peanut butter (or almond butter)

- 1 ripe banana

- 1 tablespoon of cacao nibs (for extra chocolate flavor)

- Ice cubes (optional)

- Sweetener (such as dates or agave nectar) to taste

Instructions:

Add chocolate almond milk, vegan chocolate protein powder, peanut butter, ripe banana, and cacao nibs to a blender.

Blend until all ingredients are well combined, and the shake is creamy and chocolatey.

Add ice cubes if you prefer a colder shake and blend briefly.

Sweeten with dates or agave nectar if it's not sweet enough for your liking.

Pour into a glass and indulge in this chocolate peanut butter protein delight!

4. Vegan Tropical Protein Smoothie

Ingredients:

- 1 cup of coconut milk (canned or carton)

- 1 scoop of vegan protein powder (such as pea protein or rice protein)

- 1/2 cup of frozen pineapple chunks

- 1/2 cup of frozen mango chunks

- 1/2 ripe banana

- 1 tablespoon of chia seeds

- Ice cubes (optional)

- Sweetener (such as agave nectar or dates) to taste

Instructions:

Combine coconut milk, vegan protein powder, frozen pineapple, frozen mango, ripe banana, and chia seeds in a blender.

Blend until all ingredients are well combined and the smoothie is creamy.

Add ice cubes for a colder smoothie and blend briefly.

Sweeten with agave nectar or pitted dates if desired.

Pour into a glass and transport yourself to a tropical paradise with this protein-packed delight!

5. Vegan Coffee Protein Shake

Ingredients:

- 1 cup of chilled brewed coffee (or cold brew)

- 1 scoop of vegan coffee-flavored protein powder

- 1 ripe banana

- 1 tablespoon of almond butter (or cashew butter)

- 1/2 teaspoon of cinnamon

- Ice cubes (optional)

- Sweetener (such as maple syrup or dates) to taste

Instructions:

Combine chilled brewed coffee, vegan coffee protein powder, ripe banana, almond butter, and cinnamon in a blender.

Blend until all ingredients are thoroughly combined and the shake is creamy with a coffee kick.

Add ice cubes for extra chill and blend briefly.

Sweeten with maple syrup or pitted dates if you prefer a sweeter shake.

Pour into a glass and enjoy your energizing coffee protein shake!

6. Vegan High-Protein Green Detox Smoothie

Ingredients:

- 1 cup of unsweetened almond milk (or any plant-based milk)

- 1 scoop of vegan protein powder (such as hemp protein or spirulina protein)

- 1 cup of kale leaves (stems removed)

- 1/2 cucumber

- 1/2 lemon (juiced)

- 1 tablespoon of fresh ginger (peeled and grated)

- 1 tablespoon of chia seeds

- Ice cubes (optional)

- Sweetener (such as agave nectar or dates) to taste

Instructions:

Combine almond milk, vegan protein powder, kale, cucumber, lemon juice, grated ginger, and chia seeds in a blender.

Blend until all ingredients are well combined, and the smoothie is a vibrant green color.

Add ice cubes for a refreshing twist and blend briefly.

Sweeten with agave nectar or pitted dates if you prefer a sweeter taste.

Pour into a glass and enjoy this green detox smoothie packed with protein and nutrients!

7. Vegan Blueberry Protein Smoothie

Ingredients:

- 1 cup of frozen blueberries
- 1 cup of spinach leaves
- 1 scoop of vegan protein powder (such as pea protein or hemp protein)
- 1 tablespoon of almond butter (or sunflower seed butter)
- 1 cup of almond milk (or any plant-based milk)
- 1 tablespoon of flaxseeds
- Ice cubes (optional)
- Sweetener (such as agave nectar or dates) to taste

Instructions:

Combine frozen blueberries, spinach leaves, vegan protein powder, almond butter, almond milk, flaxseeds, and ice cubes in a blender.

Blend until all ingredients are well combined, and the smoothie is a beautiful shade of blue.

Sweeten with agave nectar or pitted dates if desired.

Pour into a glass and savor this nutritious and antioxidant-rich blueberry protein smoothie!

8. Vegan Oatmeal Protein Smoothie

Ingredients:

- 1 cup of cooked and cooled oats

- 1 scoop of vegan protein powder (such as brown rice protein or soy protein)

- 1 ripe banana

- 1 cup of almond milk (or any plant-based milk)

- 1 tablespoon of almond butter (or cashew butter)

- 1/2 teaspoon of ground cinnamon

- Ice cubes (optional)

- Sweetener (such as maple syrup or dates) to taste

Instructions:

Combine cooked oats, vegan protein powder, ripe banana, almond milk, almond butter, ground cinnamon, and ice cubes in a blender.

Blend until all ingredients are thoroughly combined and the smoothie is creamy.

Sweeten with maple syrup or pitted dates if you prefer a sweeter taste.

Pour into a glass and enjoy this hearty and filling oatmeal protein smoothie!

9. Vegan Chocolate Mint Protein Shake

Ingredients:

- 1 cup of unsweetened almond milk (or any plant-based milk)

- 1 scoop of vegan chocolate protein powder

- 1/2 ripe avocado

- 1/4 teaspoon of peppermint extract

- 1 tablespoon of cacao powder (unsweetened)

- Ice cubes (optional)

- Sweetener (such as agave nectar or dates) to taste

Instructions:

Combine almond milk, vegan chocolate protein powder, ripe avocado, peppermint extract, cacao powder, and ice cubes in a blender.

Blend until all ingredients are well combined and the shake is creamy with a refreshing minty-chocolate flavor.

Sweeten with agave nectar or pitted dates if desired.

Pour into a glass and indulge in this chocolate mint protein shake!

10. Vegan Protein-Packed Banana Split Smoothie

Ingredients:

- 1 ripe banana

- 1 scoop of vegan protein powder (such as vanilla or mixed berry flavor)

- 1 cup of mixed berries (strawberries, blueberries, raspberries)

- 1 tablespoon of almond butter (or peanut butter)

- 1 cup of almond milk (or any plant-based milk)

- Ice cubes (optional)

- Toppings: sliced strawberries, cacao nibs, shredded coconut (optional)

Instructions:

Combine ripe banana, vegan protein powder, mixed berries, almond butter, almond milk, and ice cubes in a blender.

Blend until all ingredients are thoroughly combined, and the smoothie is creamy.

Pour into a glass and top with sliced strawberries, cacao nibs, and shredded coconut for a delightful banana split-inspired treat.

Enjoy your protein-packed banana split smoothie!

These high-protein vegan smoothie recipes offer a range of flavors and ingredients to keep your taste buds satisfied while providing essential nutrients and protein for your body. Enjoy these delicious and nutritious smoothies!

Baking with Protein Powder: Adding Nutritional Value to Your Treats

Baking with protein powder has become increasingly popular as more people seek ways to incorporate additional protein into their diets while enjoying their favorite baked goods. Whether you're a fitness enthusiast looking to boost your protein intake or simply want to make your treats more nutritious, protein powder can be a versatile and tasty addition to your baking endeavors.

One of the primary benefits of using protein powder in baking is the ability to increase the protein content of your recipes without significantly altering the taste or texture of the final product. Protein powder comes in various flavors, including vanilla, chocolate, and berry, allowing you to match it with your recipes' flavor profiles. This versatility means you can create protein-packed cookies, muffins, pancakes, and more while still enjoying the delicious flavors you love.

When incorporating protein powder into your baking, it's essential to choose a high-quality product that aligns with your dietary preferences. Look for protein powders that are free from artificial additives, sweeteners, and fillers. Vegan protein powders, such as those made from pea, rice, hemp, or soy protein, are available for those following plant-based diets. Whey protein powder is another popular choice for those who consume dairy products.

To get started with baking using protein powder, you can replace a portion of the flour in your recipes with protein powder. A general guideline is to replace up to one-quarter of the flour with protein powder. For example, if a recipe calls for 1 cup of flour, you can use 3/4 cup of flour and 1/4 cup of protein powder. Adjust the ratio based on your taste preferences and the type of protein powder you're using.

In addition to adding protein, protein powder can contribute a pleasant texture to baked goods. It can make cookies chewier, pancakes fluffier, and muffins more moist. However, be mindful not to overdo it, as excessive protein powder can lead to dry or dense results. Experimentation and adaptation are key to achieving the desired texture in your baked treats.

When baking with protein powder, consider the liquid content of your recipes. Protein powder can absorb liquid, so you may need to adjust the amount of liquid in your recipes to maintain the desired consistency. This may involve adding more milk or water to prevent your baked goods from becoming too dry.

Furthermore, be cautious with the type and brand of protein powder you choose, as different brands and types may have varying textures, flavors, and absorption rates. It's advisable to start with a small amount and gradually increase the protein powder in your recipes as you become familiar with its effects on your baked goods.

In conclusion, baking with protein powder offers an excellent way to add nutritional value to your treats while preserving their delicious taste and texture. By choosing the right protein powder and experimenting with recipes, you can create protein-packed baked goods that support your dietary goals and satisfy your cravings for something sweet or savory. So, get creative in the kitchen and enjoy the benefits of baking with protein powder!

Cooking Savory Dishes: Elevating Flavor and Nutrition

Cooking savory dishes is an art that allows you to create flavorful and satisfying meals that appeal to your taste buds while providing essential nutrients for your body. Savory dishes are known for their rich, hearty flavors, and they often feature ingredients like vegetables, proteins, herbs, and spices. Whether you're a seasoned chef or a novice in the kitchen, here are some tips to help you master the art of cooking savory dishes.

1. Ingredient Selection: The foundation of any savory dish lies in the quality and selection of ingredients. Fresh vegetables, lean proteins, aromatic herbs, and high-quality spices are essential. When possible, choose seasonal and locally sourced ingredients for optimal flavor and nutrition.

2. Building Layers of Flavor: Savory dishes often rely on layering flavors to create depth. Start by sautéing aromatics like onions, garlic, and ginger in oil or butter. These aromatic ingredients release their flavors and form the base of many savory recipes. As you cook, add herbs and spices at different stages to enhance the dish's complexity.

3. Protein Options: Savory dishes can feature various proteins, including poultry, beef, pork, seafood, and plant-based options like tofu, tempeh, or legumes. Properly cooking proteins, whether by roasting, grilling, or simmering, is crucial to achieving the desired texture and taste.

4. Balanced Seasoning: Achieving the right balance of salt, pepper, and other seasonings is key to a successful savory dish. Taste as you go and adjust seasonings accordingly. Remember that some ingredients, like soy sauce or miso, can add both saltiness and umami flavor to your dishes.

5. Sauces and Broths: Sauces and broths are often used to tie savory dishes together. Stocks, gravies, and reductions can add richness and moisture to dishes. Experiment with different sauces and broths to find the ones that complement your ingredients best.

6. Cooking Techniques: Explore various cooking techniques to bring out the best in your savory dishes. Techniques like roasting, braising, sautéing, and simmering offer different flavors and textures. The choice of technique depends on the ingredients and the final outcome you desire.

7. Fresh Herbs and Spices: Fresh herbs and spices play a significant role in enhancing the flavors of savory dishes. Experiment with a wide range of herbs, such as basil, thyme, rosemary, and cilantro, and spices like cumin,

coriander, paprika, and turmeric to create unique flavor profiles.

8. Presentation: The visual appeal of a savory dish is essential. Consider how you plate and garnish your creations. Fresh herbs, citrus zest, or a drizzle of high-quality olive oil can elevate the presentation and add a final burst of flavor.

9. Experimentation: Don't be afraid to experiment with new ingredients, flavors, and cuisines. Trying out different recipes and techniques allows you to expand your culinary skills and discover new savory dishes that you love.

10. Enjoy the Process: Cooking savory dishes can be a rewarding and enjoyable experience. Embrace the process, savor the aromas, and take pride in creating meals that delight your palate and those of your loved ones.

Cooking savory dishes is a delightful journey of flavors, textures, and creativity. Whether you're preparing a comforting stew, a spicy curry, or a savory pie, these tips will help you master the art of savory cooking and create dishes that leave a lasting impression. So, don your apron, gather your ingredients, and embark on your culinary adventure!

Making Protein-Rich Snacks: Nourishing and Satisfying Your Hunger

Protein-rich snacks are a great way to curb hunger, maintain energy levels, and support muscle recovery throughout the day. Whether you're looking for post-workout options or simply want to make healthier snack choices, creating protein-packed snacks can be both convenient and delicious.

1. Nuts and Seeds: Nuts like almonds, walnuts, and cashews, as well as seeds like chia, flax, and pumpkin seeds, are natural sources of protein. Create a trail mix with a variety of nuts and seeds for a satisfying and portable snack. You can also make nut butter spreads or energy bars for a quick protein boost.

2. Greek Yogurt: Greek yogurt is a protein powerhouse that can be enjoyed on its own or as a base for various snacks. Add fresh berries, honey, and a sprinkle of granola for a parfait, or blend it into a smoothie for a creamy and protein-rich treat.

3. Hummus: Hummus, made from chickpeas, is not only rich in protein but also provides fiber and healthy fats. Pair it with carrot sticks, cucumber slices, or whole-grain crackers for a satisfying and savory snack.

4. Hard-Boiled Eggs: Hard-boiled eggs are a convenient and portable source of protein. Sprinkle them with a

pinch of salt and pepper or make deviled eggs for a flavorful snack option.

5. Edamame: Edamame, young soybeans, is a protein-packed snack that can be steamed or boiled and sprinkled with sea salt. They make a delicious and nutritious finger food.

6. Cottage Cheese: Cottage cheese is a versatile protein source that can be enjoyed sweet or savory. Top it with pineapple chunks and a drizzle of honey for a sweet option or pair it with diced tomatoes and a sprinkle of black pepper for a savory twist.

7. Protein Smoothies: Blend your favorite plant-based or whey protein powder with almond milk, fruits, and a handful of spinach for a nutrient-dense smoothie. Protein smoothies are ideal for post-workout refueling.

8. Jerky: Jerky made from lean meats like turkey, beef, or chicken is a portable and protein-rich snack. Look for low-sodium options for a healthier choice.

9. Quinoa Salad: Quinoa is a complete protein and can be used to create a variety of savory or sweet snacks. Try making a quinoa salad with vegetables, herbs, and a lemon vinaigrette for a satisfying and nutritious option.

10. Tofu or Tempeh Bites: Marinate cubes of tofu or tempeh in your favorite sauce, then bake or pan-fry until crispy. These bites are not only high in protein but also offer a satisfying texture.

11. Protein Bars: Store-bought or homemade protein bars can be a convenient and customizable snack option. You can control the ingredients and flavors to suit your taste preferences.

12. Cheese and Whole Grains: Pairing cheese with whole-grain crackers or whole wheat bread can provide a balanced snack with both protein and fiber. Opt for lower-fat cheese varieties for a healthier choice.

Creating protein-rich snacks doesn't have to be complicated. With a little planning and creativity, you can prepare snacks that are not only delicious but also provide the essential protein your body needs. Whether you're on the go or relaxing at home, these protein-packed snacks will keep you nourished and satisfied throughout the day.

Meal Planning and Scheduling: Nourishing Your Body and Lifestyle

Meal planning and scheduling are essential aspects of maintaining a balanced and healthy diet while fitting into your daily routine. By strategically organizing your meals, you can ensure that you meet your nutritional needs, manage portion sizes, and make healthier food choices. Here are some tips and strategies for effective meal planning and scheduling.

1. Set Clear Goals: Begin by defining your dietary goals and objectives. Are you aiming for weight loss, muscle gain, improved energy levels, or simply a healthier diet? Understanding your goals will guide your meal planning decisions.

2. Create a Weekly Menu: Plan your meals for the week ahead. Start with breakfast, lunch, dinner, and snacks. Having a structured menu in place reduces the likelihood of impulsive, less healthy food choices.

3. Include Variety: Incorporate a variety of foods into your meal plan to ensure you get a wide range of nutrients. Include fruits, vegetables, lean proteins, whole grains, and healthy fats in your meals.

4. Portion Control: Be mindful of portion sizes. Use measuring cups or a food scale if necessary to accurately portion out your food. This helps prevent overeating and supports your dietary goals.

5. Cook in Batches: Prepare larger quantities of certain meals, such as soups, stews, or grains, and store them in individual portions. This can save time and ensure you have healthy options readily available when you're busy.

6. Plan for Snacks: Include nutritious snacks in your meal plan to keep your energy levels stable throughout the day. Healthy snacks like fruit, yogurt, nuts, or hummus with veggies can curb hunger between meals.

7. Be Mindful of Timing: Schedule your meals and snacks at consistent times throughout the day. This helps regulate your metabolism and prevents extreme hunger that can lead to unhealthy eating choices.

8. Listen to Your Body: Pay attention to hunger and fullness cues. Eat when you're hungry, but also practice portion control and avoid eating when you're not genuinely hungry.

9. Adapt to Your Lifestyle: Tailor your meal planning to your daily schedule. If you have a busy day ahead, prepare simple and portable meals. On less hectic days, you can experiment with more elaborate recipes.

10. Preparing for Special Occasions: Plan ahead for special occasions or social gatherings. If you know you'll be dining out, review the menu in advance and choose healthier options. Alternatively, eat a small, balanced meal before heading out to avoid overindulging.

11. Stay Hydrated: Don't forget about hydration. Include water, herbal teas, or infused water in your meal plan to stay adequately hydrated throughout the day.

12. Adjust as Needed: Be flexible with your meal plan and willing to adjust it if necessary. Life can be unpredictable, and sometimes you may need to adapt your meals to accommodate unexpected events or changes in your routine.

13. Seek Professional Guidance: If you have specific dietary needs or health concerns, consider consulting a registered dietitian or nutritionist. They can help you create a personalized meal plan tailored to your individual goals and requirements.

Meal planning and scheduling are valuable tools for achieving and maintaining a healthy and balanced diet. By taking a thoughtful and structured approach to your meals, you can better nourish your body, manage your weight, and enjoy the benefits of a nutritious diet that aligns with your lifestyle and goals.

Protein Needs for Active Vegans

Protein needs for active vegans are a crucial aspect of maintaining a healthy and balanced diet that supports their physical activity levels and overall well-being. Whether you're an athlete, a fitness enthusiast, or simply someone who leads an active lifestyle, ensuring an adequate intake of protein is essential for muscle repair, recovery, and sustained energy. Here are some key considerations for meeting your protein needs as an active vegan.

First and foremost, it's essential to dispel the myth that vegans struggle to obtain enough protein. There are plenty of plant-based protein sources available that can provide the necessary amino acids to support muscle growth and repair. Legumes like beans, lentils, and chickpeas, as well as tofu, tempeh, seitan, and edamame, are excellent sources of plant-based protein.

Variety in your diet is key to meeting protein needs. Different plant-based protein sources offer various amino acid profiles, so consuming a mix of these foods ensures that you obtain a wide range of essential amino acids. Incorporating a diverse selection of fruits, vegetables, grains, nuts, and seeds into your meals helps balance your protein intake.

When calculating your protein requirements, consider your level of physical activity. Active individuals typically require more protein to support muscle maintenance and recovery. A general guideline is to aim for around 1.2 to 2.2 grams of protein per kilogram of body weight per day, depending on the intensity and duration of your workouts.

Timing your protein intake can be beneficial for active individuals. Consuming protein-rich meals or snacks both before and after exercise can help optimize muscle protein synthesis and enhance recovery. Including a source of protein in your post-workout meal or snack, such as a protein shake or a tofu stir-fry, can support muscle repair and growth.

Incorporating protein-rich snacks into your daily routine can help you meet your protein needs. Options like vegan protein bars, trail mix with nuts and seeds, or a handful of almonds can provide a convenient protein boost between meals.

Keep an eye on your total calorie intake, especially if you're physically active and looking to maintain or achieve specific fitness goals. Ensuring that you're consuming enough calories from a variety of plant-based sources helps provide the energy necessary to fuel your workouts and support your protein needs.

Supplementing with plant-based protein powders can be a practical way to meet your protein requirements, especially on days when it's challenging to obtain enough protein through whole foods alone. There are various vegan protein powders available, such as pea protein, hemp protein, rice protein, and more, which can be added to smoothies or used in recipes.

Lastly, remember that a well-balanced diet is essential for overall health and performance. Alongside protein, ensure that you're getting an adequate intake of carbohydrates, healthy fats, vitamins, and minerals to support your active lifestyle.

In conclusion, active vegans can meet their protein needs through a well-planned and diverse plant-based diet. By including a variety of protein-rich foods, paying attention to timing, and considering supplementation when necessary, active vegans can support their physical activity levels while maintaining a healthy and nutritious diet.

Performance Enhancement with Protein Supplements

Performance enhancement with protein supplements has become a common practice among athletes, bodybuilders, and individuals engaged in various forms of physical activity. Protein is a crucial macronutrient that plays a fundamental role in muscle repair, growth, and overall recovery. While it's possible to obtain adequate protein from whole foods, protein supplements offer convenience, versatility, and precise control over protein intake, making them a valuable tool for those seeking to optimize their performance.

One of the primary benefits of protein supplements is their ability to deliver a concentrated dose of protein quickly. This can be particularly advantageous for athletes and active individuals who need to meet their protein needs efficiently, especially in the post-workout period when muscles are most receptive to protein intake. Protein supplements in the form of shakes, powders, or bars can be rapidly absorbed and utilized by the body.

Whey protein, derived from milk, has long been a popular choice among athletes due to its high-quality protein content and rapid digestion. However, for vegans and those with lactose intolerance, plant-based protein supplements like pea protein, rice protein, hemp protein, and others offer equally effective options. These plant-based alternatives provide the necessary amino acids for muscle recovery without the use of animal products.

Protein supplements can also help individuals fine-tune their macronutrient intake. Athletes and bodybuilders often have specific protein requirements to support their training goals, and supplements allow them to easily adjust their protein intake to meet these needs. This precision can be especially valuable when following strict dietary regimens or participating in weight-based sports.

Additionally, protein supplements can be integrated into various culinary creations. They can be blended into smoothies, incorporated into baked goods, or used as a base for protein-rich snacks. This versatility allows athletes and fitness enthusiasts to enjoy a variety of flavors and textures while still meeting their protein goals.

It's important to note that while protein supplements can enhance performance and recovery, they should not be relied upon as the sole source of protein in one's diet. Whole foods such as lean meats, fish, tofu, legumes, and dairy products provide a wide range of essential nutrients, including vitamins, minerals, and fiber, that are essential for overall health.

For individuals considering protein supplements, it's advisable to consult with a registered dietitian or nutritionist who can provide personalized recommendations based on specific fitness goals and dietary preferences. Additionally, individuals with underlying health conditions should exercise caution and seek professional guidance when incorporating supplements into their diet.

In conclusion, protein supplements offer a practical and effective means of enhancing performance and supporting muscle recovery for athletes and active individuals. Whether

Case Studies of Vegan Athletes

Case studies of vegan athletes provide compelling insights into the capacity of plant-based diets to support athletic performance and overall health. While the notion of thriving as an athlete on a vegan diet was once met with skepticism, these real-life examples showcase the success and achievements of individuals who have adopted plant-based eating patterns.

One noteworthy case is that of Scott Jurek, a renowned ultramarathoner and multiple-time winner of the Western States Endurance Run. Jurek transitioned to a vegan diet during his running career and credits it with improving his recovery times and endurance. His accomplishments, including setting an Appalachian Trail speed record, demonstrate the potential for plant-based nutrition to fuel extraordinary feats of athleticism.

Another compelling example is Patrik Baboumian, a professional strongman and former Germany's Strongest Man. Baboumian's plant-based journey began in 2011 when he adopted a vegan diet. Despite initial doubts about maintaining his strength, he has continued to break records and win competitions as a vegan athlete. His feats, such as setting a world record for the yoke walk, highlight the capacity of plant-based diets to support muscle growth and power.

In the world of professional sports, tennis player Venus Williams has garnered attention for her vegan lifestyle. Williams, diagnosed with an autoimmune disease, shifted to a raw vegan diet to manage her health. She has not only sustained her professional tennis career but also achieved remarkable success, including Grand Slam titles, while embracing plant-based nutrition.

Additionally, Olympic weightlifter Kendrick Farris embraced veganism to improve his health and athletic performance. Farris represented the United States in three Olympic Games and set American records in weightlifting while following a plant-based diet. His achievements demonstrate that plant-based nutrition can adequately fuel strength and power sports.

Brendan Brazier, a former professional Ironman triathlete and two-time Canadian 50km Ultra Marathon Champion, has followed a vegan diet for years and has credited it with improving his recovery, endurance, and overall athletic performance. He is also the creator of the Vega line of plant-based nutritional products, further emphasizing the compatibility of veganism and athletic achievement.

Another noteworthy case is that of Fiona Oakes, an accomplished marathon runner and ultramarathoner. Oakes is not only a vegan athlete but also an advocate for animal welfare. She holds multiple marathon course records, including the Antarctic Ice Marathon, and has completed numerous challenging ultramarathons. Her achievements highlight the capacity of a plant-based diet to support long-distance running and endurance sports.

David Carter, a former NFL defensive lineman, is another compelling example of a vegan athlete. Carter transitioned to a plant-based diet for health reasons, citing the significant improvements in his recovery, energy levels, and overall well-being. Despite the physical demands of professional football, he maintained his strength and performance while advocating for the benefits of plant-based nutrition.

Dotsie Bausch, an Olympic silver medalist in cycling, also embraced veganism during her athletic career. She discovered that a plant-based diet improved her cardiovascular health, endurance, and recovery. Bausch's success at the highest level of competitive cycling demonstrates the potential of vegan nutrition to support aerobic sports and cardiovascular health.

These case studies collectively challenge the notion that animal products are necessary for athletic performance and recovery. These athletes have not only thrived on a vegan diet but have also achieved remarkable success in their respective sports. Their experiences underscore the importance of balanced nutrition, proper meal planning, and informed dietary choices in optimizing plant-based diets for athletes.

Vegan Protein for Children

Ensuring an adequate intake of vegan protein for children is essential to support their growth, development, and overall health. While animal products are traditional sources of protein, a well-planned vegan diet can provide all the necessary protein and nutrients children need for optimal growth and vitality.

Legumes, including beans, lentils, and chickpeas, are excellent sources of plant-based protein and can be incorporated into various child-friendly dishes such as bean burritos, lentil soup, or hummus with veggie sticks. These foods not only provide protein but also essential fiber, vitamins, and minerals.

Tofu and tempeh are soy-based products that offer a versatile and protein-rich addition to a child's diet. Tofu can be blended into smoothies, added to stir-fries, or used to make kid-friendly dishes like crispy tofu nuggets.

Tempeh can be crumbled and used as a protein-rich topping for pasta or salads.

Nuts and seeds are another valuable source of vegan protein. Nut butters, such as peanut or almond butter, can be spread on whole-grain bread or used as dips for fruit slices. Seeds like chia, flax, and hemp can be added to oatmeal, yogurt, or baked goods to boost protein content.

Whole grains like quinoa, brown rice, and oats not only provide carbohydrates but also contain decent amounts of protein. They can be the foundation for nourishing meals such as quinoa and vegetable stir-fry or oatmeal topped with nuts and berries.

Plant-based milk alternatives, such as almond milk, soy milk, or oat milk, are often fortified with protein and essential nutrients. These can be used in cereal, smoothies, or as a beverage alongside meals to ensure children receive the necessary nutrients for growth.

Fruits and vegetables also contribute to a child's protein intake, although they are not as protein-dense as other plant foods. However, they provide essential vitamins, minerals, and antioxidants that are crucial for overall health and should be included in a balanced vegan diet.

Supplements like vitamin B12, iron, and omega-3 fatty acids may be necessary for vegan children, as these nutrients can be more challenging to obtain from plant-based sources alone. Consultation with a pediatrician or registered dietitian can help ensure that children receive appropriate supplements if needed.

It's crucial to be mindful of portion sizes and variety in a child's vegan diet to ensure they receive an adequate and well-rounded intake of protein and essential nutrients. Monitoring their growth and development, along with regular check-ups, can help parents and caregivers gauge the effectiveness of their child's diet.

Providing vegan protein for children is achievable through a well-balanced and diverse diet that includes legumes, tofu, tempeh, nuts, seeds, whole grains, plant-based milk, fruits, and vegetables. By carefully planning meals and monitoring their nutritional intake, parents can support their children's growth and development while adhering to a vegan lifestyle that aligns with ethical and environmental values.

Pregnancy and Breastfeeding

Pregnancy and breastfeeding are critical phases in a woman's life that demand special attention to nutrition and dietary choices. It's essential to provide the body with the right nutrients to support the health of both the mother and the developing baby during pregnancy and breastfeeding. Vegan mothers can maintain a vegan lifestyle while ensuring they meet their nutritional needs and support the growth and development of their child.

Protein is a vital component of a vegan diet during pregnancy and breastfeeding. Pregnant and breastfeeding women require more protein to support the growth of the fetus or infant and to meet their own increased metabolic needs. Vegan protein sources include legumes, tofu, tempeh, nuts, seeds, and whole grains. Including a variety of these foods in daily meals can help ensure an adequate protein intake.

Calcium is crucial for the development of the baby's bones and teeth. While dairy products are the most common source of calcium, vegans can obtain this mineral from fortified plant-based milk, calcium-set tofu, leafy green vegetables (like kale and collard greens), almonds, tahini, and calcium-fortified foods. Ensuring a consistent intake of these calcium-rich foods is essential for vegan mothers.

Iron is another nutrient of concern during pregnancy, as the body's iron needs increase to support the growth of the placenta and fetus. Plant-based sources of iron include lentils, beans, tofu, spinach, and fortified cereals. Consuming vitamin C-rich foods, like citrus fruits and bell peppers, alongside iron-rich foods can enhance iron absorption.

Vitamin B12 is crucial for brain development, and vegan mothers must ensure they get an adequate supply during pregnancy and breastfeeding. While B12 is primarily found in animal products, vegans can obtain it from fortified foods, such as plant-based milk, breakfast cereals, and nutritional yeast. Vitamin B12 supplements are also recommended during pregnancy and breastfeeding to ensure sufficient intake.

Folate, or folic acid, is essential for preventing birth defects and supporting the baby's neural tube development. Vegan sources of folate include leafy greens, lentils, beans, and fortified foods like cereals and bread. Many prenatal supplements also contain adequate folate levels.

Omega-3 fatty acids, particularly DHA (docosahexaenoic acid), play a crucial role in fetal brain and eye development. Vegans can obtain DHA from algae-based supplements, which provide a plant-based source of this essential nutrient.

A well-balanced vegan diet, rich in whole grains, fruits, vegetables, legumes, nuts, and seeds, can provide the necessary nutrients during pregnancy and breastfeeding. However, consulting with a healthcare provider or registered dietitian is advisable to ensure that nutrient needs are met. Regular prenatal check-ups and blood tests can monitor the mother's nutritional status and the baby's development to address any deficiencies promptly.

Aging Vegans

Aging vegans, like anyone in the aging population, have unique nutritional considerations to maintain their health and well-being as they grow older. While a well-balanced vegan diet can provide essential nutrients, aging individuals must pay extra attention to certain aspects of their diet to ensure they meet their changing nutritional needs.

Protein remains crucial for aging vegans, as it supports muscle mass and strength, especially as muscle loss tends to occur with age. Vegan sources of protein, including legumes, tofu, tempeh, nuts, seeds, and plant-based protein powders, should be included in meals to ensure an adequate intake. Protein consumption should be distributed throughout the day to optimize muscle protein synthesis.

Calcium is vital for maintaining bone health, which becomes increasingly important as individuals age. Vegan sources of calcium, such as fortified plant-based milk, calcium-set tofu, leafy green vegetables, almonds, and tahini, should be a regular part of the diet to support bone density.

Vitamin B12 absorption can decrease with age, so it's crucial for aging vegans to continue monitoring their B12 intake and possibly increase supplementation if needed. Vitamin B12 deficiency can lead to neurological issues and cognitive decline, which are concerns in the aging population.

Omega-3 fatty acids, particularly EPA (eicosapentaenoic acid) and DHA (docosahexaenoic acid), play a role in brain health and may help reduce the risk of cognitive decline. Vegan sources of these essential fatty acids include algae-based supplements, flaxseeds, chia seeds, and walnuts. Integrating these foods into the diet can support cognitive function in aging vegans.

Fiber-rich foods like fruits, vegetables, whole grains, and legumes continue to be essential for digestive health. Adequate fiber intake can help prevent constipation and support gastrointestinal well-being, which can become more of a concern with age.

Antioxidants found in colorful fruits and vegetables, such as berries, spinach, and broccoli, are valuable for combating oxidative stress and reducing the risk of chronic diseases associated with aging, including heart disease and certain cancers.

Maintaining proper hydration is critical for aging individuals, as dehydration can lead to a range of health issues. Drinking enough water and consuming hydrating foods like fruits and vegetables can help prevent dehydration.

Supplementation of specific nutrients, such as vitamin D and calcium, may be recommended for aging vegans to support bone health. Consulting with a healthcare provider or registered dietitian can help determine individualized supplement needs based on dietary intake and health status.

Regular exercise is essential for aging vegans to support muscle strength, bone density, and overall mobility. Combining a well-balanced diet with physical activity can contribute to a healthier and more active aging process.

Health Conditions and Dietary Restrictions

Food allergies and intolerances are essential considerations for anyone with dietary restrictions, including vegans. Allergies or intolerances to common vegan foods like nuts, soy, or gluten may require careful label reading and the selection of suitable substitutes. It's essential to communicate dietary needs when dining out or purchasing packaged vegan foods to avoid allergenic ingredients.

Celiac disease, a condition triggered by gluten consumption, demands strict adherence to a gluten-free diet. While many vegan foods are naturally gluten-free, individuals with celiac disease must still be vigilant about cross-contamination and choose certified gluten-free grains, such as rice, quinoa, and oats. Gluten-free baking and cooking often involve alternative flours and starches.

Diabetes management on a vegan diet involves monitoring carbohydrate intake, as carbohydrates significantly affect blood sugar levels. Vegan diabetics may choose complex carbohydrates with a low glycemic index and monitor portion sizes. Balancing carbohydrate intake with dietary fiber, healthy fats, and plant-based protein sources is essential for blood sugar control.

Hypertension, or high blood pressure, can be managed on a vegan diet through careful attention to sodium intake. Processed and high-sodium vegan foods should be limited, while an emphasis on fruits, vegetables, whole grains, lean plant-based proteins, and low-sodium seasonings can help maintain blood pressure within a healthy range.

Individuals with heart disease, including high cholesterol and atherosclerosis, often adopt a vegan diet to reduce the risk of cardiovascular complications. A heart-healthy vegan diet focuses on minimizing saturated and trans fats, added sugars, and sodium while emphasizing unsaturated fats, dietary fiber, and omega-3 fatty acids from plant-based sources like flaxseeds, walnuts, and fatty fish alternatives.

Religious or cultural dietary restrictions, such as kosher or halal practices, require individuals to adhere to specific food preparation and ingredient guidelines. While veganism is compatible with these restrictions, careful attention to sourcing, preparation, and consumption of foods is necessary to ensure compliance with religious or cultural dietary laws.

Vegans, whether motivated by ethical, environmental, or health reasons, should consider specific nutrients when planning their diet. Key nutrients of concern for vegans include protein, vitamin B12, iron, calcium, and omega-3 fatty acids. Careful selection of plant-based protein sources, fortified foods, and supplements may be necessary to meet these nutritional needs.

Debunking Common Vegan Protein Myths:

Myth 1: Vegans can't get enough protein.

Truth: Protein is abundantly available in plant-based foods. Legumes like lentils, chickpeas, and beans, as well as tofu, tempeh, seitan, and nuts, are rich sources of plant-based protein. By including a variety of these foods in their diets, vegans can easily meet their protein needs.

Myth 2: Plant-based protein is incomplete.

Truth: While some plant-based protein sources may lack certain essential amino acids, a well-balanced vegan diet that includes a variety of foods provides all the necessary amino acids. Complementary protein sources, such as rice and beans or peanut butter on whole-grain bread, can ensure amino acid balance.

Myth 3: Animal protein is superior to plant protein.

Truth: Both animal and plant proteins offer essential amino acids. Plant-based proteins often come with additional health benefits like fiber, antioxidants, and lower saturated fat content, making them a valuable part of a healthy diet.

Myth 4: Vegans need to combine proteins at every meal.

Truth: Protein combining, or the concept of eating specific combinations of plant foods at each meal, is unnecessary. As long as vegans consume a variety of protein-rich foods throughout the day, they will obtain all the essential amino acids they need.

Myth 5: You have to eat large amounts of protein to meet your needs.

Truth: Protein needs vary depending on factors like age, activity level, and overall health. Most people can meet their protein needs by consuming a well-balanced diet without excessive protein intake. Excess protein is not necessarily beneficial and may have health risks.

Myth 6: Plant-based athletes can't build muscle or perform well.

Truth: Numerous vegan athletes excel in various sports, debunking the myth that animal protein is necessary for athletic performance. Proper meal planning and adequate protein intake can support muscle growth and athletic achievements on a vegan diet.

Myth 7: Plant-based protein sources lack variety.

Truth: The variety of plant-based protein sources is extensive, from legumes, grains, and nuts to tofu, tempeh, and plant-based protein powders. Vegans can enjoy a diverse range of protein-rich foods in their diet.

Myth 8: Plant-based protein is less digestible.

Truth: While plant-based proteins may have different digestion rates compared to animal proteins, they are still highly digestible when properly prepared and consumed as part of a balanced diet.

Complete vs. Incomplete Proteins Myths and Misconceptions:

Myths and misconceptions about complete vs. incomplete proteins have caused confusion about protein sources in diets, particularly for those following plant-based or vegan lifestyles. Here, we debunk some common myths:

Myth 1: Incomplete proteins are low-quality proteins.

Truth: Incomplete proteins, which lack one or more essential amino acids, are often mistakenly considered low-quality. In reality, they can be rich sources of nutrients and offer various health benefits. Legumes, grains, nuts, seeds, and vegetables are examples of incomplete protein sources, and when consumed in a balanced diet, they provide all essential amino acids.

Myth 2: Animal proteins are always complete.

Truth: While animal proteins typically contain all essential amino acids, not all animal protein sources are equal. Some animal-based foods, like gelatin and certain cuts of meat, are lower in certain amino acids. Additionally, processed and high-fat animal products may not be the healthiest sources of complete protein.

Myth 3: You must combine proteins in the same meal for completeness.

Truth: The concept of combining complementary protein sources at every meal is a common myth. The body stores amino acids and combines them as needed, so there's no need for meticulous protein combining at every meal. Eating a varied diet of plant-based foods throughout the day naturally provides complete protein.

Myth 4: Plant-based diets are deficient in complete proteins.

Truth: Plant-based diets can easily meet protein needs when individuals consume a diverse range of foods. Legumes, tofu, tempeh, quinoa, and soy products are examples of complete plant-based protein sources. Including these foods in a balanced vegan diet ensures adequate protein intake.

Myth 5: Quinoa is the only complete plant-based protein.

Truth: Quinoa is an excellent complete plant-based protein source, but it's not the only one. Soy products like tofu and tempeh, as well as seitan and some legumes like soybeans, provide complete protein. Including a variety of these foods in the diet ensures all essential amino acids are met.

Myth 6: Incomplete proteins are lacking in protein content.

Truth: Incomplete protein sources, like grains and legumes, are not low in protein. They can be rich in protein and other essential nutrients. While they may be lower in specific amino acids, combining them with a variety of other plant-based protein sources ensures a well-rounded and adequate protein intake.

Myth 7: Incomplete proteins are not as nutritious.

Truth: Incomplete protein sources are often nutrient-dense and provide essential vitamins, minerals, and fiber. Incorporating them into a balanced diet offers various health benefits, including improved heart health and digestion.

Vegan Protein and Muscle Building Myths and Misconceptions:

Myths and misconceptions about vegan protein and muscle building have caused confusion among those seeking to build muscle on a plant-based diet. Here, we debunk some common myths:

Myth 1: Vegan diets lack sufficient protein for muscle building.

Truth: Vegan diets can provide plenty of protein for muscle building. Legumes, tofu, tempeh, seitan, lentils, and plant-based protein powders are excellent sources of plant-based protein that can support muscle growth. Proper meal planning ensures adequate protein intake for vegan muscle builders.

Myth 2: Plant-based protein is inferior to animal protein for muscle growth.

Truth: Plant-based protein is not inferior to animal protein for muscle building. Both types of protein contain essential amino acids necessary for muscle synthesis. Vegans can meet their protein needs and build muscle effectively by consuming a variety of plant-based protein sources.

Myth 3: You need to eat more protein as a vegan to build muscle.

Truth: While protein needs may vary based on factors like activity level and goals, excessively high protein intake is not necessary for muscle building. Vegan athletes and bodybuilders can achieve their protein needs through balanced meals and may benefit from spreading protein intake throughout the day.

Myth 4: Vegan bodybuilders can't get enough essential amino acids.

Truth: Vegan diets can provide all essential amino acids when individuals consume a diverse range of plant-based foods. Combining protein sources, such as beans and rice or hummus and whole-grain pita, ensures a complete amino acid profile and supports muscle protein synthesis.

Safety and Potential Side Effects

Ensuring Safe Consumption:

While vegan protein sources offer numerous health benefits, it's essential to ensure their safe consumption. This includes proper food handling, storage, and preparation. Adequate cooking, especially for legumes and grains, helps eliminate potential foodborne pathogens and enhance digestibility. Additionally, using clean cooking utensils and maintaining good hygiene practices when preparing vegan protein-rich foods is crucial for safe consumption.

Allergies and Sensitivities:

Individuals may have allergies or sensitivities to certain plant-based protein sources. Common allergens among vegans include nuts, soy, and gluten-containing grains. It's essential to be aware of allergens and carefully read food labels to avoid allergenic ingredients. In cases of known allergies or sensitivities, selecting alternative protein sources can help prevent adverse reactions while maintaining a balanced vegan diet.

Digestive Issues:

Some individuals may experience digestive issues when consuming certain plant-based proteins. Beans, lentils, and cruciferous vegetables like broccoli and cauliflower can sometimes lead to gas and bloating due to their fiber content. To minimize these issues, gradually introducing these foods into the diet and cooking them thoroughly can improve digestibility. Fermented plant-based foods like tempeh and miso may also be better tolerated by some individuals.

Overconsumption Risks:

While plant-based diets are generally healthful, overconsumption of certain vegan protein sources can pose risks. High intake of soy-based products, for example, may lead to excessive consumption of isoflavones, which could have hormonal effects. Maintaining a balanced diet that incorporates a variety of protein sources helps mitigate the risk of overconsumption of specific nutrients or compounds.

Safety and potential side effects related to vegan protein consumption are essential considerations when following a plant-based diet. Ensuring safe food handling and preparation, being mindful of allergies and sensitivities, addressing digestive issues with proper cooking techniques, and avoiding overconsumption of specific foods are key aspects of maintaining a healthy and well-rounded vegan diet. By paying attention to these factors, individuals can enjoy the benefits of vegan protein sources while minimizing potential side effects.

The Environmental Impact of Plant-Based Protein

The environmental impact of plant-based protein sources is a significant consideration when evaluating the sustainability of dietary choices. Plant-based proteins are generally associated with lower environmental impacts compared to animal-based protein sources. Here are some key aspects of the environmental impact of plant-based protein:

Lower Greenhouse Gas Emissions: Plant-based protein sources, such as legumes, grains, and vegetables, typically have a lower carbon footprint than animal-based proteins. Livestock farming, particularly cattle, is a major contributor to greenhouse gas emissions due to methane production, deforestation for pastureland, and the energy-intensive process of raising animals for food. Choosing plant-based proteins helps reduce these emissions.

Reduced Land Use: Producing plant-based proteins generally requires less land than animal agriculture. Crops used for plant-based protein can be grown more efficiently, using fewer resources and less land area. This helps conserve natural habitats and reduces the pressure to clear forests for agricultural purposes.

Lower Water Footprint: The water footprint of plant-based protein sources is typically lower than that of animal-based proteins. Livestock farming demands substantial water resources for drinking, feed production, and cleaning. In contrast, growing crops for plant-based proteins is generally less water-intensive. Choosing plant-based proteins can help reduce water scarcity and improve water conservation efforts.

Reduced Deforestation: Animal agriculture is a leading driver of deforestation in various regions worldwide. Clearing forests for cattle ranching or to grow feed crops contributes to biodiversity loss and disrupts ecosystems. Opting for plant-based proteins supports efforts to combat deforestation and protect natural habitats.

Lower Energy Consumption: Producing plant-based proteins is generally more energy-efficient than raising animals for meat and dairy. Plant-based agriculture requires fewer resources like fossil fuels for transportation, as well as reduced energy input for maintaining animals. Lower energy consumption contributes to a more sustainable food system.

Reduced Pollution: Livestock farming can lead to environmental pollution through the release of manure and chemicals into waterways. The concentration of animals in factory farms can exacerbate these issues. Plant-based protein production typically generates fewer pollutants and has a lower impact on local ecosystems.

Preservation of Biodiversity: Choosing plant-based proteins helps preserve biodiversity by reducing the pressure on ecosystems caused by agriculture expansion. The loss of biodiversity can have negative consequences for ecosystem stability, resilience, and the provision of essential ecosystem services.

Sustainable Farming Practices: Many plant-based protein sources, such as legumes, can be grown using sustainable farming practices like crop rotation and reduced pesticide use. These practices promote soil health and reduce the reliance on synthetic chemicals.

Plant-based proteins generally have a lower environmental impact compared to animal-based proteins. By choosing plant-based protein sources, individuals can contribute to reducing greenhouse gas emissions, conserving land and water resources, preventing deforestation, and promoting more sustainable and environmentally friendly food production practices. These choices play a crucial role in mitigating the environmental challenges associated with food production.

Ethical Considerations

Ethical considerations play a central role in the decision to adopt a vegan diet or consume plant-based proteins. For many individuals, ethical concerns are a primary motivation for choosing plant-based foods. Here are some key ethical considerations associated with veganism and plant-based diets:

Animal Welfare: One of the primary ethical motivations for adopting a vegan diet is concern for animal welfare. Many people choose to abstain from animal products to avoid contributing to the suffering and exploitation of animals in the food industry. Factory farming practices, which often involve crowded and unsanitary conditions, as well as practices like debeaking and tail docking, are sources of significant ethical concern.

Cruelty-Free Living: Vegans aim to live a cruelty-free lifestyle by avoiding products and practices that involve animal testing or the use of animals for entertainment, clothing, or other purposes. This commitment extends beyond diet to encompass choices related to cosmetics, clothing, and entertainment.

Environmental Ethics: Environmental considerations are closely linked to ethics. Many individuals adopt plant-based diets due to concerns about the environmental impact of animal agriculture, including deforestation, habitat destruction, water pollution, and greenhouse gas emissions. By reducing their reliance on animal products, they aim to minimize their contribution to these environmental issues.

Global Food Security: Some ethical perspectives emphasize the importance of addressing global food security and equitable resource distribution. Plant-based diets can be seen as a way to use agricultural resources more efficiently, potentially reducing hunger and addressing ethical concerns related to food access.

Sustainability: Sustainability is a key ethical consideration in the context of plant-based diets. Ethical vegans often argue that transitioning to plant-based agriculture is a more sustainable way to feed the growing global population while minimizing resource depletion and ecological harm.

Health Ethics: For some, ethical considerations also extend to personal health. Choosing plant-based foods may align with an ethical commitment to one's own well-being, including reducing the risk of chronic diseases and promoting overall health.

Supporting Ethical Food Systems: Ethical vegans may choose plant-based diets to support alternative food systems that prioritize sustainability, animal welfare, and fair labor practices. This includes supporting local, organic, and cruelty-free food production.

Cultural and Religious Ethics: In some cultures and religions, ethical considerations related to diet are deeply ingrained. Certain religious or cultural beliefs may prohibit the consumption of specific animal products, leading individuals to adopt plant-based diets as a reflection of their ethical values.

Ethical Consumerism: Ethical considerations extend beyond diet to encompass broader consumer choices. Ethical consumers aim to support companies and products that align with their values, which may include those related to animal welfare, sustainability, and social justice.

In conclusion, ethical considerations are a driving force behind the adoption of vegan diets and the consumption of plant-based proteins. Individuals who prioritize animal welfare, environmental sustainability, equitable resource distribution, and personal health often find alignment with plant-based and vegan lifestyles as a way to live in accordance with their ethical values. These considerations shape their dietary choices and broader lifestyle decisions.

The Future of Vegan Protein Sustainability

The future of vegan protein sustainability holds great promise as it responds to the growing awareness of environmental, ethical, and health concerns. Technological advancements are set to revolutionize the landscape, with innovations like plant-based meat alternatives and cellular agriculture creating sustainable and realistic meat alternatives that cater to a broader audience. These innovations not only reduce the environmental footprint but also make it more appealing for consumers to transition to sustainable protein sources.

Diversification of protein sources is expected to be a key trend, moving beyond traditional options like soy and legumes. Researchers and food producers are exploring novel plant-based protein sources, including fungi, algae, and microorganisms, offering unique nutritional profiles and sustainability benefits. These emerging sources expand the possibilities for sustainable protein production.

The adoption of sustainable farming practices will continue to gain importance in the cultivation of plant-based protein sources. Methods such as regenerative agriculture, organic farming, and agroforestry enhance soil health, reduce pesticide use, and minimize environmental impact. These practices align with the principles of sustainability and ethical food production, ensuring that the future of vegan protein remains environmentally responsible.

Supporting local and small-scale producers of vegan proteins is another avenue for promoting sustainability. By reducing the carbon footprint associated with transportation, this approach contributes to regional food systems' growth while ensuring access to sustainable protein sources. Farmers' markets, community-supported agriculture (CSA), and direct-to-consumer sales of plant-based products can strengthen local economies and enhance the sustainability of protein production.

Increasing environmental awareness among consumers is a driving force in the future of vegan protein sustainability. As individuals become more conscious of their food choices' environmental impact, they are likely to demand more sustainable vegan protein options. This demand, in turn, encourages businesses to adopt environmentally friendly practices in their production processes.

The role of policy and regulation cannot be underestimated in shaping the future of vegan protein sustainability. Governments and regulatory bodies may enact policies that encourage sustainable practices in the food industry, including plant-based protein production. These policies can further accelerate the transition towards more environmentally friendly and ethical food systems, making sustainable vegan protein an integral part of the future food landscape.

Affordable Protein Sources

Affordable protein sources are crucial for ensuring that individuals of all income levels have access to nutritious and balanced diets. Access to affordable protein is vital for maintaining overall health, especially for populations facing economic challenges. Here are some key affordable protein sources:

Legumes: Legumes, such as beans, lentils, and chickpeas, are some of the most affordable protein sources available. They are rich in protein, fiber, and essential nutrients, making them an excellent choice for budget-conscious individuals. Dried legumes are often more cost-effective than canned varieties, and buying in bulk can provide even more savings.

Grains: Whole grains like rice, oats, and quinoa are not only affordable but also provide a source of plant-based protein. They can be incorporated into a variety of dishes, from simple grain bowls to complex recipes, making them versatile options for those on a budget.

Tofu and Tempeh: While tofu and tempeh may be slightly more expensive than some other plant-based proteins, they are still affordable sources of high-quality protein. These soy-based products are known for their versatility in various recipes, allowing individuals to create budget-friendly and protein-rich meals.

Seitan: Seitan, a protein-rich meat substitute made from wheat gluten, is an economical choice for those looking to add protein to their diet. It's often used in vegan and vegetarian dishes and can be a cost-effective alternative to meat.

Eggs: For those who include eggs in their diet, they are a relatively inexpensive source of high-quality protein. Eggs are versatile and can be prepared in numerous ways, making them a budget-friendly option for many.

Canned Fish: For individuals who include seafood in their diet, canned fish like tuna and salmon can provide affordable protein. These options are shelf-stable and can be a cost-effective way to incorporate animal-based protein into meals.

Plant-Based Protein Powders: While some protein powders can be expensive, there are affordable plant-based protein powder options available. Pea protein, rice protein, and soy protein powders can be purchased at reasonable prices and added to smoothies or recipes to boost protein intake.

Frozen Vegetables: Frozen vegetables can be an economical way to increase protein intake. Options like frozen peas, spinach, and broccoli contain protein and can be included in various dishes without the risk of spoilage.

Nuts and Seeds: While nuts and seeds can be relatively more expensive, they can still be affordable when purchased in bulk. Small amounts of nuts and seeds can add protein and healthy fats to meals and snacks.

Dairy Alternatives: Some dairy alternatives, like almond milk, soy milk, and oat milk, can be affordable sources of plant-based protein. They can be used in place of cow's milk in various recipes and are often fortified with additional nutrients.

In conclusion, affordable protein sources are essential for ensuring that individuals from diverse socioeconomic backgrounds can access nutritious and protein-rich foods. By incorporating budget-friendly protein options like legumes, grains, tofu, and canned fish into their diets, individuals can maintain a healthy and balanced protein intake without breaking the bank.

Thrifty Shopping Tips

Thrifty shopping tips are essential for individuals looking to maximize their grocery budget while still obtaining nutritious and satisfying foods. Here are some effective strategies for thrifty shopping:

Plan Your Meals: Before heading to the store, plan your meals for the week. This helps you create a shopping list with only the items you need, reducing the likelihood of impulse purchases.

Use Coupons and Discounts: Look for coupons, digital deals, and discounts offered by grocery stores or online retailers. Many stores have loyalty programs that offer savings to regular customers.

Buy Generic Brands: Generic or store-brand products are often more budget-friendly than name-brand alternatives. They are typically of similar quality and can save you money over time.

Compare Prices: Pay attention to unit prices on shelves to compare the cost per ounce or pound of different products. This helps you determine which items offer the best value for your money.

Shop Sales and Clearance: Keep an eye out for sales, clearance items, and reduced-price products. These can be an excellent way to save on groceries, especially for non-perishable or frozen items.

Purchase in Bulk: Buying items in bulk can lead to significant savings over time. Look for pantry staples like rice, pasta, canned goods, and dried beans that can be purchased in larger quantities.

Limit Convenience Foods: Pre-packaged and convenience foods are often more expensive than whole ingredients. Opt for whole vegetables and fruits and prepare meals from scratch when possible to save money.

Reduce Meat Consumption: Meat is typically one of the more expensive items in a grocery bill. Consider incorporating more plant-based proteins like beans, lentils, and tofu into your diet to reduce meat expenses.

Minimize Food Waste: Be mindful of food expiration dates and try to use ingredients before they go bad. Proper storage and meal planning can help reduce food waste and save money.

Shop Seasonal Produce: Seasonal fruits and vegetables are often cheaper and fresher than out-of-season options. Plan your meals around what's in season to maximize savings.

Join a Rewards Program: Many grocery stores offer rewards programs that provide discounts and special offers to members. Signing up for these programs can lead to additional savings.

Bring a Shopping List: Stick to your shopping list and avoid purchasing items not on your list. Impulse purchases can quickly add up and strain your budget.

Limit Eating Out: Reducing the frequency of dining out or ordering takeout can significantly impact your food budget. Cooking meals at home is usually more cost-effective.

Utilize Leftovers: Make use of leftovers by incorporating them into future meals. This reduces food waste and eliminates the need to prepare entirely new dishes.

Shop Online: Online grocery shopping can provide access to exclusive discounts and offers. Additionally, it can help you avoid impulse purchases since you can review your cart before checking out.

Incorporating these thrifty shopping tips into your grocery routine can help you make the most of your budget while still enjoying nutritious and satisfying meals. With careful planning and smart choices, you can save money without sacrificing the quality of your diet.

DIY Protein Supplements

Creating your own DIY protein supplements and recipes can be a cost-effective and customizable way to meet your protein needs. Here are some ideas and recipes for making your own protein supplements and incorporating them into delicious dishes:

DIY Protein Powder:

You can make your own protein powder blend using various plant-based protein sources. Combine ingredients like dried beans, lentils, peas, and oats, then grind them into a fine powder using a high-speed blender or a food processor. This homemade protein powder can be used in smoothies, oatmeal, or baked goods.

Protein-Packed Smoothie:

Blend together a homemade protein powder with ingredients like frozen berries, banana, spinach, almond milk, and a tablespoon of nut butter for a protein-packed smoothie. Customize it with your favorite flavors and sweeteners for a nutritious and satisfying breakfast or post-workout snack.

Plant-Based Protein Bars:

Create your own protein bars by mixing your homemade protein powder with ingredients like dates, nuts, seeds, and a touch of maple syrup. Press the mixture into a baking pan, refrigerate until firm, and then cut it into bars. These homemade protein bars are perfect for on-the-go snacks.

Tofu Scramble:

Tofu is an excellent source of plant-based protein. Make a savory tofu scramble by crumbling firm tofu and sautéing it with vegetables like bell peppers, onions, and spinach. Season with turmeric, nutritional yeast, and your favorite spices for a flavorful and protein-rich breakfast.

Chickpea Salad:

Chickpeas are packed with protein and can be the base of a satisfying salad. Combine cooked chickpeas with diced cucumber, tomatoes, red onion, fresh herbs, and a simple lemon tahini dressing for a protein-packed and refreshing salad.

Lentil Soup:

Lentils are a great source of plant-based protein and can be used in various dishes. Make a hearty lentil soup by simmering brown or green lentils with vegetables, broth, and aromatic spices. Enjoy it as a warming and protein-rich meal.

Quinoa Bowl:

Quinoa is a complete protein source and can be the foundation of a nutritious bowl. Cook quinoa and top it with roasted vegetables, avocado, a protein-rich sauce like tahini or hummus, and a sprinkle of nuts or seeds for added texture and flavor.

Protein-Packed Pasta:

Choose whole-grain or legume-based pasta for an extra protein boost. Combine cooked pasta with a homemade tomato sauce loaded with lentils or chickpeas, and top it with nutritional yeast for a cheesy flavor. This protein-packed pasta dish is both satisfying and nutritious.

Homemade Protein Shakes:

Blend your homemade protein powder with ingredients like almond milk, a ripe banana, a spoonful of nut butter, and a dash of cinnamon for a delicious and protein-rich shake. You can also add spinach or kale for an extra nutrient boost.

Protein-Packed Energy Bites:

Create your own energy bites by combining your homemade protein powder with rolled oats, almond butter, honey, and a mix of nuts and dried fruits. Roll the mixture into bite-sized balls and refrigerate for a convenient and protein-rich snack.

These DIY protein supplements and recipes offer a wide range of options to incorporate plant-based protein into your diet. Experiment with different ingredients and flavors to tailor your protein sources to your preferences and dietary needs while enjoying nutritious and delicious meals and snacks.

Emerging Trends in Plant-Based Protein

Emerging trends in plant-based protein are reshaping the food industry and providing consumers with more diverse and sustainable protein options. These trends reflect growing interest in plant-based diets for health, environmental, and ethical reasons. Here are some key trends in plant-based protein:

Alternative Protein Sources: Beyond traditional plant-based protein sources like soy and legumes, there is a growing interest in exploring alternative protein sources. These include algae, fungi, microorganisms, and even insects. These novel sources offer unique nutritional profiles and can be more sustainable to produce.

Plant-Based Meat Alternatives: The rise of plant-based meat alternatives, such as burgers, sausages, and nuggets, has been a significant trend. These products closely mimic the taste and texture of meat and have gained popularity among both vegetarians and omnivores. They are increasingly available in restaurants and supermarkets.

Clean Labeling: Consumers are becoming more conscious of the ingredients in their food. Many plant-based protein products are shifting toward clean labeling, using simpler and more recognizable ingredients. This trend aligns with the demand for minimally processed foods.

Fermentation: Fermentation is being used to create plant-based proteins with improved textures and flavors. Fermented foods like tempeh and kombucha are gaining popularity, and this technology is being applied to plant-based protein production.

Customizable Plant-Based Proteins: Some companies are offering customizable plant-based protein options. Consumers can choose the source and type of protein they prefer, such as pea, rice, or hemp protein, allowing for more personalized nutrition.

Whole Plant Proteins: Instead of relying solely on isolated protein sources, there is a shift toward incorporating whole plant proteins into products. For example, snacks and energy bars include whole nuts and seeds as protein sources.

Plant-Based Seafood: As concerns about overfishing and mercury contamination grow, plant-based seafood alternatives are emerging. These products replicate the taste and texture of fish and seafood while being entirely plant-based.

Ethical Sourcing and Sustainability: Consumers are increasingly interested in the ethical and sustainability aspects of plant-based proteins. They want to know where their food comes from and how it is produced. Brands that prioritize ethical sourcing and sustainability are gaining popularity.

DIY Plant-Based Protein: Some individuals are opting to make their own plant-based protein sources at home, such as DIY protein powders made from a blend of legumes, seeds, and grains. This trend reflects a desire for more control over the ingredients used in plant-based diets.

Plant-Based Protein for Sports Nutrition: Plant-based protein is gaining traction in the sports nutrition industry. Athletes and fitness enthusiasts are recognizing the benefits of plant-based proteins for muscle recovery and overall health.

Global Plant-Based Cuisine: Plant-based diets from various cultures are gaining recognition and inspiring new culinary trends. Dishes like falafel, sushi rolls with plant-based fish, and vegan curries are becoming more accessible and celebrated.

These emerging trends in plant-based protein reflect a dynamic shift in consumer preferences and the food industry's response to the demand for sustainable, ethical, and nutritious protein sources. As technology and innovation continue to drive the development of plant-based protein products, consumers can expect even more diverse and appealing options in the future.

Innovations and Product Developments

Innovations and product developments in the plant-based protein industry are driving substantial changes in the food landscape, catering to the increasing demand for sustainable and ethical protein sources. These developments are not only reshaping consumer choices but also influencing the strategies of food companies and restaurants:

Advanced Meat Alternatives: Plant-based meat alternatives have seen remarkable advancements. Companies are continually improving their products' texture, taste, and nutritional profiles. Innovations like the use of heme to replicate the "bloody" flavor of meat or the development of plant-based chicken that mimics the fibrous texture of poultry have gained traction.

Cellular Agriculture: Cellular agriculture, also known as lab-grown or cultured meat, represents a significant innovation in the plant-based protein space. It involves growing animal cells in a lab environment to create real meat without the need for raising and slaughtering animals. This technology holds the promise of producing meat that is nearly indistinguishable from traditional animal-based meat.

Hybrid Products: Some companies are experimenting with hybrid products that combine both animal and plant-based proteins. These products aim to cater to flexitarian consumers who want to reduce their meat consumption but still enjoy the taste and texture of traditional meat.

Plant-Based Seafood: Innovations in plant-based seafood alternatives are on the rise. Companies are developing plant-based versions of popular seafood items like fish fillets, shrimp, and crab cakes. These products not only provide a sustainable option but also address concerns about overfishing and mercury contamination.

Sustainable Ingredients: Innovations in sourcing sustainable ingredients are shaping the plant-based protein industry. Companies are focusing on using environmentally friendly crops, reducing water usage, and minimizing the carbon footprint of their products. Some are even exploring the use of regenerative agriculture practices.

Plant-Based Dairy Alternatives: Beyond meat, plant-based dairy alternatives are continually evolving. Innovations in plant-based milk, cheese, and yogurt have expanded the range of choices for consumers. These products now come in a variety of flavors and textures, making them more appealing to a broader audience.

Nutritional Enhancement: Plant-based protein products are being fortified with additional nutrients to provide a more comprehensive nutritional profile. Innovations include adding vitamins, minerals, and omega-3 fatty acids to mimic the nutritional content of animal-based products.

Customization and Personalization: Some companies are offering customization options, allowing consumers to create their own plant-based protein products. This personalization trend caters to individual preferences and dietary needs, empowering consumers to tailor their protein choices.

Eco-Friendly Packaging: Innovations extend to packaging materials as well. Companies are exploring eco-friendly and sustainable packaging options to minimize waste and reduce the environmental impact of their products.

Global Culinary Influences: The plant-based protein industry is being influenced by global culinary traditions. Dishes from various cultures are inspiring new plant-based products, adding diversity and flavor to the plant-based protein market.

These innovations and product developments in the plant-based protein industry are driving a dynamic shift in the food landscape. They are not only expanding choices for consumers but also contributing to sustainability, ethical considerations, and improved nutrition. As technology and creativity continue to shape this industry, consumers can expect an even wider array of appealing and sustainable plant-based protein options in the future.

Prospects for Vegan Protein Research

The prospects for vegan protein research are promising and essential as the demand for sustainable and ethical protein sources continues to grow. Researchers are focusing on various areas to advance our understanding of vegan proteins and improve their quality, nutrition, and sustainability.

Nutritional Profiling: One key area of research is the nutritional profiling of vegan protein sources. Scientists are examining the amino acid profiles, vitamin and mineral content, and overall nutritional value of plant-based proteins to ensure they meet dietary requirements. This research is crucial for formulating well-balanced vegan diets.

Improving Protein Quality: Researchers are developing methods to enhance the protein quality of plant-based sources. This includes optimizing processing techniques, such as extrusion and fermentation, to improve protein digestibility and bioavailability. By making plant proteins more efficient sources of essential amino acids, they can better meet human nutritional needs.

Novel Protein Sources: Exploring novel protein sources beyond the traditional ones, like soy and legumes, is another focus of research. Algae, fungi, microorganisms, and even insects are being investigated as potential sustainable protein sources. These sources offer unique nutritional profiles and can be cultivated with lower environmental impact.

Clean Labeling: Researchers are working on clean labeling strategies to simplify ingredient lists and make plant-based protein products more appealing to consumers who prefer recognizable ingredients. This research involves finding natural and minimally processed alternatives to commonly used additives.

Taste and Texture: Achieving the desired taste and texture in plant-based meat and dairy alternatives is an ongoing area of research. Scientists are developing innovative approaches to replicate the sensory experiences associated with animal-based products. This includes optimizing ingredient combinations and processing methods.

Sustainability Metrics: Researchers are developing comprehensive sustainability metrics to assess the environmental impact of different plant-based protein sources and production methods. These metrics help guide consumers, policymakers, and food producers in making more sustainable choices.

Consumer Acceptance: Understanding consumer preferences and barriers to adopting plant-based proteins is critical. Research in this area involves studying consumer perceptions, behaviors, and motivations related to plant-based diets. This insight can inform marketing strategies and product development.

Food Security: Researchers are exploring how plant-based proteins can contribute to global food security by efficiently using land and resources. They are studying crop varieties and farming practices that optimize protein production while minimizing environmental impacts.

Health Benefits: Investigating the health benefits of plant-based diets is an ongoing focus. Research has shown that well-planned vegan diets can have positive effects on heart health, weight management, and the prevention of chronic diseases. Further studies are needed to explore the long-term health outcomes of plant-based eating patterns.

Policy and Regulation: Researchers are engaged in policy and regulatory discussions related to vegan proteins. This includes evaluating labeling standards, health claims, and food safety regulations to ensure that plant-based products meet quality and safety standards.

In conclusion, the prospects for vegan protein research are multifaceted and vital for addressing the challenges and opportunities in the growing plant-based protein industry. As researchers continue to explore these areas, they contribute to the development of more sustainable, nutritious, and appealing plant-based protein options, making it easier for individuals to adopt and maintain plant-based diets.

Empowering Vegans to Meet Their Protein Needs

Empowering vegans to meet their protein needs is crucial for ensuring they maintain a balanced and nutritious diet. While plant-based diets offer numerous health and environmental benefits, it's important to pay attention to protein intake, as it is a vital macronutrient for overall well-being. Here are several ways to empower vegans to meet their protein needs effectively:

1. Education and Awareness: Educate vegans about the importance of protein in their diet and the role it plays in muscle maintenance, immune function, and overall health. Raising awareness about protein-rich plant-based foods is essential for informed dietary choices.

2. Balanced Meal Planning: Encourage vegans to plan well-balanced meals that include protein-rich foods like legumes, tofu, tempeh, seitan, nuts, seeds, and whole grains. A varied and balanced diet ensures a diverse intake of essential amino acids.

3. Knowledge of Protein Sources: Familiarize vegans with a wide range of plant-based protein sources. Understanding which foods are rich in protein allows

them to make informed choices and incorporate variety into their diet.

4. Protein-Rich Snacking: Promote the consumption of protein-rich snacks like nuts, seeds, edamame, and plant-based yogurt. These options can help vegans maintain steady energy levels throughout the day.

5. Cooking Skills: Empower vegans with cooking skills that allow them to prepare delicious and protein-packed meals at home. Cooking with plant-based protein sources can be both economical and rewarding.

6. Protein Supplements: In some cases, protein supplements like pea, rice, or hemp protein powders may be useful for vegans, especially athletes or those with high protein requirements. Educate them on how to choose high-quality supplements and incorporate them into their diet if needed.

7. Proper Food Pairing: Teach vegans about food pairing to create complete protein sources. Combinations like rice and beans, peanut butter on whole-grain bread, or hummus with pita bread provide complementary amino acids.

8. Nutritional Tracking: Encourage the use of nutritional tracking apps or journals to monitor protein intake. These tools can help vegans ensure they are meeting their daily protein requirements.

9. Seek Professional Guidance: When necessary, recommend consulting with a registered dietitian or nutritionist who specializes in plant-based diets. These experts can provide personalized guidance and meal plans tailored to individual needs.

10. Supportive Community: Foster a supportive community where vegans can exchange tips, recipes, and experiences related to meeting their protein needs. Peer support can be valuable for individuals transitioning to or maintaining a vegan lifestyle.

11. Recipe Resources: Provide access to recipe resources and cookbooks specifically focused on plant-based protein-rich dishes. Creative and flavorful recipes can make it enjoyable for vegans to incorporate protein into their meals.

Empowering vegans to meet their protein needs involves a combination of education, resources, and support. By arming them with knowledge, culinary skills, and a variety of protein sources, individuals can thrive on a plant-based diet while ensuring they meet their protein requirements for optimal health and well-being.

Encouragement for a Healthy, Sustainable Lifestyle

Embracing a healthy and sustainable lifestyle is a significant step toward personal well-being and environmental stewardship. While the journey may present challenges, it's essential to remember that every small effort contributes to positive change. Here's some encouragement for those pursuing a healthier and more sustainable way of life.

Making sustainable choices in daily life, such as reducing waste, conserving energy, and choosing eco-friendly products, can have a substantial collective impact on the environment. Recognize that every conscious decision to reduce, reuse, or recycle matters, and it inspires others to follow suit.

Incorporating more plant-based foods into your diet is not only beneficial for your health but also for the planet. You're making a meaningful difference by reducing the demand for animal agriculture, which is a significant contributor to greenhouse gas emissions and deforestation. Each plant-based meal is a step towards a more sustainable future.

Exercise and physical activity are essential components of a healthy lifestyle. They not only improve physical fitness but also boost mental well-being. Remember that every workout, whether it's a brisk walk, a yoga session, or a gym session, contributes to your overall health and vitality.

Exploring local and seasonal foods can be an exciting culinary journey. It supports local farmers, reduces food miles, and connects you with your community. Seek out farmers' markets and local producers to discover fresh, seasonal ingredients that enhance your meals.

Mental health is an integral part of a healthy lifestyle. Taking time for self-care, mindfulness, and stress reduction is vital. Embrace practices like meditation, deep breathing exercises, or simply spending time in nature to nurture your mental well-being.

Celebrate your progress and small victories along the way. Whether it's successfully completing a challenging workout, preparing a delicious plant-based meal, or reducing your household waste, each accomplishment brings you closer to a healthier and more sustainable lifestyle.

Share your journey with friends and family. Your enthusiasm and positive changes can inspire those around you to embark on their path to a healthier and more sustainable life. Encourage open conversations about sustainability and well-being within your social circles.

Remember that setbacks are a natural part of any journey. Don't be discouraged by occasional slip-ups or challenges. Use them as opportunities to learn and grow, and then get back on track with renewed determination.

Embracing a healthy and sustainable lifestyle is a meaningful and rewarding endeavor. It not only benefits your well-being but also contributes to the well-being of the planet and future generations. Every effort, no matter how small, makes a positive impact, and your journey inspires others to join in creating a healthier and more sustainable world.

www.ingramcontent.com/pod-product-compliance
Lightning Source LLC
Chambersburg PA
CBHW050730260726
48661CB00001B/151